Intravenous Therapy Administration
A practical guide

Nicola Brooks

Illustrated by Rachy McKenzie

Intravenous Therapy Administration: A practical guide
Nicola Brooks

ISBN: 978-1-905539-90-1

First published 2017

British Library Cataloguing in Publication Data
A catalogue record for this book is available from the British Library

Notice

Clinical practice and medical knowledge constantly evolve. Standard safety precautions must be followed, but, as knowledge is broadened by research, changes in practice, treatment and drug therapy may become necessary or appropriate. Readers must check the most current product information provided by the manufacturer of each drug to be administered and verify the dosages and correct administration, as well as contraindications. It is the responsibility of the practitioner, utilising the experience and knowledge of the patient, to determine dosages and the best treatment for each individual patient. Any brands mentioned in this book are as examples only and are not endorsed by the publisher. Neither the publisher nor the authors assume any liability for any injury and/or damage to persons or property arising from this publication.

To contact M&K Publishing write to:
M&K Update Ltd · The Old Bakery · St. John's Street
Keswick · Cumbria CA12 5AS
Tel: 01768 773030 · Fax: 01768 781099
publishing@mkupdate.co.uk
www.mkupdate.co.uk

Designed and typeset by Mary Blood
Printed in Scotland by Bell & Bain, Glasgow

Full the full range of M&K Publishing books please visit our website:
www.mkupdate.co.uk

Contents

Preface

Intravenous Therapy Administration – A Practical Guide is a simple 'pick up, put down' resource for any healthcare practitioner who needs to carry out intravenous therapy. This book provides the basic underlying theory and underpinning knowledge you need, using a step-by-step approach to offer guidance in how to administer intravenous fluids and medicines. It will be equally helpful, whether you are already practising intravenous therapy and wish to refresh or update your knowledge or you are learning this skill for the first time.

Intravenous Therapy Administration – A Practical Guide is split into short, simple chapters, making it very easy to use. Each chapter contains intended learning outcomes, clinical points for practice, and activities that enable the reader to relate the content to their own clinical area.

Chapter 1 discusses administration of intravenous therapy, giving reasons for its use and identifying its benefits and disadvantages. Adequate knowledge of the circulatory system is essential prior to undertaking administration of intravenous therapy. Chapter 2 therefore provides an overview of the circulatory system, and discusses the relevant anatomy and physiology of the peripheral vascular system. Chapter 3 builds on Chapter 2 by focusing on different types of intravenous access, and considering appropriate care and site management. Chapter 4 discusses the calculation of medication doses, and provides activities to enable healthcare practitioners to update their knowledge of relevant medication calculations used in the administration of intravenous fluid or medication.

Chapter 5 focuses on how medications work, and describes relevant pharmacodynamics and pharmacokinetics. Chapter 6 looks at safe administration techniques used in the administration of intravenous fluids and medications, and demonstrates a step-by-step approach to enable the healthcare practitioner to prepare and administer intravenous therapy safely. Chapter 7 looks at the use of infusion devices to support the safe administration techniques discussed in the previous chapter. Chapter 8 focuses on the risks, complications and adverse reactions associated with intravenous therapy. Finally, Chapter 9 explores the professional responsibilities of the healthcare practitioner.

Note: As a healthcare practitioner, you must always ensure that you are familiar with your own healthcare provider's policies and procedures, in addition to using this resource.

About the author

Nicola Brooks is a Senior Lecturer in Adult Nursing at De Montfort University, Leicester, and a Registered Nurse (Adult). She undertook her Diploma in Higher Education (Nursing) (Dip HE) and qualified as a nurse in 1995.

Following registration, Nicola has obtained a wealth of experience in surgical nursing, working across surgical specialities such as Colo-rectal, Ear, Nose and Throat, Plastic Surgery and Breast Care. Nicola has also spent some time working within the acute Surgical Admissions Unit and Primary Care. Having completed her BSc (Hons) in Healthcare Practice, Nicola moved to work within Higher Education, where she completed her Master's in Education, and has spent time teaching undergraduate students clinical skills, surgical care and professional development issues on the pre-registration BSc (Hons) Nursing programme.

Nicola maintains her links with clinical practice, and maintains her clinical credibility by working in the acute setting. She is also the author of *Venepuncture and Cannulation: A Practical Guide*, 2nd edition (M&K Publishing 2017).

Acknowledgements

This book is dedicated to my family – in particular, Paul, Luca, Lara and my mum. You are all 'my rock' and my world. Thank you for always being there, looking out for me, and for providing me with endless love and support to allow me to do this.

Special thanks also go to my 'work family' who in crazy times keep me sane and provide lots of love, laughter and energy when I need it most. I am blessed to work with such an amazing team who always make me smile and give me strength to get through!

Cormac Norton (Senior Lecturer) has been a star and written the second chapter of this book for me. Cormac's clinical background is in emergency medicine and nurse prescribing. I am so grateful for his contribution. I also need to extend my endless thanks to Rachy McKenzie who has drawn the illustrations for this book as well as *Venepuncture and Cannulation*. Rachy has the ability to translate my ideas and (very rough) drawings into something amazing! For that, I am truly grateful.

Nicola Brooks

Chapter 1

What is intravenous therapy and why is it used?

Learning outcomes

At the end of this chapter, the practitioner will be able to:

- **Understand what intravenous therapy is**
- **Recognise the different methods of administering intravenous therapy**
- **Identify the advantages and disadvantages of intravenous therapy.**

What is intravenous therapy?

Intravenous (IV) therapy is the administration of medicines or fluids directly into a patient's vein. For IV therapy to commence, the patient will need to have a vascular access device inserted. This is a piece of equipment that provides access to the patient's vascular system (Gabriel 2008). Vascular access is typically provided either through a central venous catheter (CVC) or a peripheral vascular access device (PVAD). A CVC is a thin, flexible tube that is used to administer medicines, fluids or blood products over a long period of time. It is inserted in the arm or chest, through the skin, into a large vein. A PVAD is described as 'a plastic tube inserted into a peripheral vein' (Boyd 2013), and is commonly known as a cannula. Manufacturers use the term Venflon, which is a brand name.

Insertion of a CVC or PVAD will allow direct access into the circulatory system (the bloodstream) so that the patient can receive the IV therapy required – for example, IV fluids, medications or the transfusion of blood or blood products. The administration of IV therapies is commonplace within healthcare practice (Lavery 2010), and this procedure is viewed as a central part of the healthcare practitioner's role and responsibilities. IV therapy is now an important aspect of medicines management; it is widely used in healthcare settings, particularly within the hospital environment.

Why has the use of IV therapy grown?

The procedure and practice of IV therapy has grown rapidly since it was broadly described in the late 1960s to early 1970s, primarily due to the benefits it offers. Figures taken from as far back as the 1990s show that a high percentage of hospitalised patients received IV therapy at some point during their stay (Workman 1999). Even in the early 2000s, it was recognised that up to 60% of patients admitted to hospital were likely to receive intravenous therapy via an intravenous (IV) device (Wilson 2001). This number continues to rise today.

Against a background of increasing demand for hospital beds and lengthening waiting lists, IV therapy has the advantage that it can be provided within the patient's home, as an alternative to hospitalisation (O'Hanlon *et al.* 2008). Many community healthcare services now offer an IV therapy service, as a strategy to avoid hospital admission for patients with long-term conditions, or (alternatively) to avoid repeated hospital visits. Medical problems that have been successfully treated with IV therapy within the home environment include cellulitis and urinary tract infections as well as bone and joint infections (O'Hanlon *et al.* 2008).

Why use IV therapy?

There are many reasons why the intravenous route may be used, in preference to other medication administration methods. These include situations where:

- Blood or blood products need to be transfused
- Fluids or electrolytes need to be replaced or maintained
- A rapid response is required (e.g. in an emergency, when medication needs to be administered quickly)
- An oral route may be inappropriate (e.g. due to nausea and vomiting, patient being nil by mouth pre- or post-operatively, or patient being unconscious)
- Medication cannot be given intra-muscularly because of the risk of bleeding (e.g. HIV patients and haemophiliac patients)
- It is necessary to achieve a high, predictable level of medication within the circulation (e.g. a septic patient)

- It is necessary to administer a medication as an infusion, as this allows an individual titrated dose to be administered
- The medication itself cannot be absorbed orally (e.g. Vancomycin or Gentamycin)
- The medication is destroyed by stomach acid (e.g. when insulin or heparin is administered).

Activity 1.1

Why is IV therapy used in your own clinical setting? Is it the most appropriate route of administration? If not, can you identify reasons why this method is currently being used?

How is IV therapy administered?

IV therapy can be administered using the following methods:

- Bolus administration (e.g. the administration of medicines using a small volume of fluid, administered within a 5-minute timeframe)
- Intermittent infusion (e.g. the administration of medicines or the transfusion of blood/ blood products, typically delivered in a period between 5 minutes and 24 hours)
- Continuous infusion (e.g. the transfusion of fluid when the patient is unable to tolerate sufficient volumes of oral fluid over longer than a 24-hour period).

What are the advantages and disadvantages of IV therapy?

IV therapy is a complex area of medicines management, and it is not without potential risk of serious harm for the patient (Lavery & Ingram 2008). There are many advantages to using an intravenous approach, as summarised in Table 1.1 (below). However, the benefits should always outweigh the risks for both the patient and the healthcare practitioner. The healthcare practitioner will need to undertake a thorough assessment of the patient's condition prior to using the IV route.

The practitioner will also need to ensure that they are competent, and possess the skill and knowledge required, to administer IV therapy safely. They will need to undertake additional training to equip them for this role, as well as being assessed as competent in their practice. Specific training requirements will be discussed in more detail in Chapter 9.

Table 1.1 The benefits and risks of IV therapy

Benefits	Risks
Intravenous administration allows administration of a medicine when the oral route cannot be used (e.g. for a patient that is nil by mouth or has acute nausea and vomiting, or due to disease processes).	There is an increased risk of administration hazards, such as phlebitis, speed shock, infiltration and extravasation.
There is a quick response, as administration of intravenous medicines avoids the absorption phase.	There is a risk of fluid overload (when using the intermittent or continuous infusion options). This is a particular risk if large volumes of fluids are used and if the rate of administration is not controlled.
Bolus administration does not overload the patient with fluid (e.g. if the patient is fluid restricted).	There is a risk of medication errors when working out the rate of infusion (for intermittent or continuous infusions).
Bolus or intermittent infusion is ideal if the medication if not chemically stable enough for a continuous route to be used.	There is an extra cost to purchase equipment and IV fluids, as these are additional resources.
Continuous infusions allow a constant blood level to be maintained, and therefore produce a constant effect.	There is an increased risk of bacterial growth as a result of the duration of the intravenous infusion.
	It is difficult or impossible to reverse the dose and its action.
	The patient could potentially suffer an allergic reaction or anaphylaxis.
	There is a risk of systemic complications (e.g. sepsis, air embolism or catheter fragment embolism).

Activity 1.2

Now that you have gained an understanding of intravenous therapy, and identified some of the reasons why intravenous therapy may be used, make sure that you read your local healthcare provider's policy and

procedure on the preparation and administration of intravenous fluids and medications. Check that you have understood and adopted the working practices detailed in your local guidelines before undertaking this role.

Possible complications of IV therapy

Administering intravenous fluid or medication can potentially be dangerous for patients. The speed of the infusion given will require close monitoring, and the patient should also be carefully observed. General additional factors will need to be considered, such as:

- If a patient is at risk (e.g. in cardiac failure), use an infusion pump (see Chapter 7 for specific guidance on using infusion pumps).
- If you are using a gravity feed, use a drip rate formula to monitor the infusion rate.
- Watch the PVAD (cannula) closely. If a device is placed near a joint, they can be 'positional'. If a patient moves that specific area of the body, the rate of the infusion may be quickly altered.
- Patients may inadvertently 'tamper' with the infusion to make it go through more quickly. In this case, there is a risk of harm to the patient.
- All infusions require constant monitoring, and the patient's vital signs will need to be closely observed (Boyd 2013).

Summary

This chapter has provided a broad introduction to intravenous therapy, considering what it is and why it may be used. The risks and benefits of using an intravenous route have also been identified.

Chapter 2

An overview of the circulatory system, and related anatomy and physiology of the peripheral vascular system

Cormac Norton

Learning outcomes

At the end of this chapter, the practitioner will be able to:

- **Discuss the structure of the circulatory system**
- **Have a basic understanding of the anatomy and physiology of the peripheral vascular system**
- **Identify the structural differences between an artery and a vein**
- **Identify the most common anatomical sites for venepuncture and cannulation.**

Introduction

It is important to have a good knowledge of anatomy and physiology and to understand how the circulatory system works. This chapter will provide a brief overview; you may wish to read a dedicated anatomy and physiology text if you require more detailed information.

The human circulatory system has three key components:

● The heart
● Blood
● Blood vessels.

The heart

The heart is a four-chambered pump. The heart's pumping action can appear confusing. It may be helpful to separate functions to the right and left side of the heart.

Table 2.1 Right-side heart functions

● Deoxygenated blood is delivered to the *right atrium* by two of the largest veins in the body – the inferior and superior venae cavae.
● The *right atrium* pumps blood to the *right ventricle*.
● The *right ventricle* pumps blood to the lungs for oxygenation via the *pulmonary artery*.

The right side of the heart contains two of the heart's four chambers – the right atrium and ventricle. The primary role of the right side is to pump deoxygenated blood to the lungs (Nair & Peate 2013). Deoxygenated blood enters the right side of the heart. From there, it travels to the lungs.

At this point it is useful to highlight one of the key differences between arteries and veins: Arteries carry blood **away** from the heart; veins carry blood **back** to the heart.

You will notice from the description above that the venae cavae (large veins) are carrying blood *back* to the heart, while the pulmonary *artery* carries blood away from the heart. Once blood has been oxygenated, it takes the following journey from the lungs to the left side of the heart and on to the rest of the body:

Table 2.2 Left-side heart functions

● Once blood has been oxygenated in the lungs it is carried back to the *left atrium* via the *pulmonary vein*.
● The *left atrium* pumps blood into the *left ventricle*.
● The *left ventricle* is the most powerful chamber of the heart and pumps blood via the *aorta* (the largest artery in the body).

- The *aorta* carries blood to the rest of body through a network of arteries (Nair & Peate 2013).

Blood

Blood is essential for life and has many functions within the human body. The three key functions are:

1. Transport: Blood carries oxygen, glucose, electrolytes and other nutrients to cells to enable functioning of those cells. Waste products from those cells (such as carbon dioxide) are carried away by the blood for elimination.

2. Defence: Cells in the blood play a vital role in the body's immune system. These 'defensive cells' include white cells and antibodies. The blood can also coagulate, forming clots and scabs. This helps prevent further injury to the body from fluid loss.

3. Maintenance of homeostasis: Blood also enables the body to manage temperature and the pH (balance of acid and alkali within the body). Homeostasis is a complex process, in which blood plays a vital part.

Blood first travels away from the heart via the aorta (an artery). Gradually, as the blood travels through the network of arteries, the arteries become narrower, and eventually they become arterioles. These arterioles enter tissue and continue to branch out and reduce in size as they do so.

The arterioles then branch into tiny vessels called capillaries. At this point, the exchange of materials occurs. For example, oxygen will leave the blood and enter the cell, and waste products will leave the cells and enter the blood (Nair & Peate 2013).

The blood now begins its journey back to the heart. As the capillaries leave the tissue, they become venules. As the vessels continue, they increase in size, becoming veins. Finally, all the veins converge into the vena cava, returning the blood to the right side of the heart (Nair & Peate 2013).

Understanding the differences between an artery and a vein

Apart from the functional differences between an artery and a vein discussed above, there are some structural differences that are important in relation to the insertion of a peripheral vascular access device (PVAD).

Both arteries and veins consist of three layers of tissue:

- The outermost layer: The Tunica Externa, which gives support and stability
- The middle layer: The Tunica Media, which allows for changing blood flow and pressure
- The innermost layer: The Tunica Intima, which facilitates blood flow.

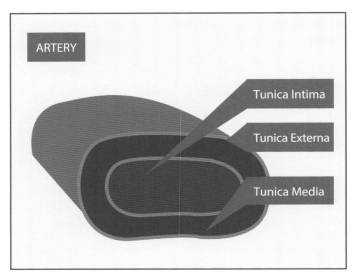

Figure 2.1 The structure of the artery

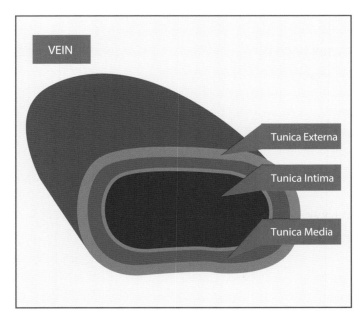

Figure 2.2 The structure of the vein

Arteries are designed to withstand blood travelling at relatively high pressure (such as 120mmHg). Veins carry blood at a much lower pressure – for example, around 80mmHg.

The key structural difference between an artery and a vein is the Tunica Media. In arteries, this middle layer consists of thick, elastic, muscular tissue. This enables arteries to expand and respond quickly to a rise in pressure in the vessel. This elasticity allows an artery to propel blood as it travels from the heart (Tortora & Derrickson 2011).

Activity 2.1

To identify the difference between veins and arteries, feel for the radial artery in your wrist on the palm side of your hand (about 5cm below the base of your thumb).

If you roll your index and middle fingers over the artery, you will feel a round, yet elastic 'tube' beneath your fingers. You will feel the pulsations through the artery. This pulsation is caused by the artery expanding in response to blood pumped by the left ventricle. The artery contracts, ensuring that the blood can continue to the hand.

If you move your fingers towards the centre of your wrist, you will feel a very rigid structure travelling from your elbow to your hand. This is a tendon. This feels solid, does not pulsate and moves when you move your fingers.

Turn your hand around and let it hang by your side. You should be able to see the veins on the back of your hand become more prominent. Gently feel the most prominent of these veins. Although they feel round, they cannot withstand significant pressure and will go 'flat' quite easily. The vein has no pulsation.

Veins do not have as robust and muscular a middle layer. In contrast, the Tunica Externa is much thicker than an artery. This allows veins to expand, but they are not elastic like arteries, and therefore cannot pulsate in the same manner. When blood pressure is reduced, it may still be possible to feel (palpate) arteries. However, veins appear to collapse and may be impossible to palpate.

One further structural difference that is relevant to inserting a PVAD is that veins have valves, whereas arteries do not. These valves ensure that blood flows in one direction to assist with venous return.

Related anatomy of the peripheral vascular system

Bones, although not functionally relevant to the insertion of a PVAD, serve as useful landmarks to identify an appropriate site. In the forearm, the radius extends from the elbow to just below the thumb. It can be palpated at the prominence known as the radial styloid, just proximal to the thumb. It can also be palpated towards the elbow until it is barely palpable below the bradioradialis muscle in the forearm to its origin at the radial head as part of the elbow. This bone lends its name to both the radial artery and radial nerve. To find the radial pulse, simply palpate on the palmar side of the radial styloid.

Likewise, the ulna can be palpated very easily and lends its name to both the ulnar artery and nerve. The ulnar nerve can be palpated on the palmar side of the ulnar styloid, and the ulnar nerve lies very close to this structure. Nerves and arteries are commonly found directly adjacent to each other, forming a neurovascular bundle

The elbow is formed from three bones – the radius, the ulna and the humerus. The radius and ulna form the lower arm, and the humerus forms the upper arm. If the arm is held with the palm of the hand facing forwards (facing the ceiling), the anterior surface of the elbow (the area facing uppermost), when relaxed, forms a natural dip. This is known as the antecubital fossa, and, although not ideal, it is a common site for a PVAD.

Summary

In this chapter, we have learnt that it is essential to have an adequate knowledge of the circulatory system and the structure of veins and arteries. A detailed knowledge of the structure and location of veins will support the healthcare practitioner in the safe administration of intravenous fluids and medications.

Chapter 3

Intravenous access and care of the site

Learning outcomes

At the end of this chapter, the practitioner will be able to:

- **Identify the different ways of delivering intravenous therapy**
- **Understand what central venous catheters are and their importance in intravenous therapy**
- **Care for a central venous catheter safely and effectively**
- **Understand how to place a peripheral vascular access device**
- **Care for a peripheral vascular access device safely and effectively.**

How is intravenous therapy delivered?

Intravenous (IV) therapy can be administered in a variety of ways. The most common is by means of a peripheral venous access device (PVAD), otherwise known as a cannula. A PVAD is a short-term, temporary device that is usually inserted into the veins of the forearm or the hand (Hindley 2004).

If there is difficulty gaining venous access, an alternative is to use a central venous catheter (CVC). CVC is an umbrella term for a line placed into a large vein, known as a central line or central venous line. A CVC can be placed into a large vein leading to the heart, into the neck (internal jugular vein), chest (subclavian vein or axillary vein), or through large veins in the arm. In this case it is also known as a peripherally inserted central catheter (PICC) line.

The femoral vein (in the groin) should be avoided, because there is a higher associated risk of deep vein thrombosis and catheter-related infection compared to the internal jugular or subclavian veins (Loveday *et al.* 2014). CVCs are typically inserted for longer-term IV access. A CVC is simply a soft hollow plastic tube that can be left in place for any period from a few weeks to a few months (though any such device should always be removed immediately if it is no longer required).

What are CVCs used for?

CVCs are used to administer medication or fluids that cannot be taken by mouth or, in the case of IV therapy, administer fluids or medications that would harm a smaller peripheral vein. CVCs are commonly used for:

- Administration of long-term IV antibiotics or parenteral nutrition
- Chemotherapy administration
- IV therapy when peripheral intravenous access is impossible
- Administration of medicines that cause phlebitis if given peripherally through a peripheral access device, e.g. amioderone, calcium chloride, potassium and dopamine.

What are the advantages of using CVCs?

Using a CVC has many advantages, as it can also allow for rapid administration of fluid (e.g. for a patient who is in shock). In addition, some CVCs have more than one channel (known as a lumen), which allows for different medications to be administered at the same time, without the medicines mixing together. Some medications (such as adrenaline, dopamine and amioderone) can only be administered centrally, as they cause vasoconstriction in veins.

CVCs generally have the following features:

- Soft, hollow tubes that may be separated into two or three different channels (called lumens)
- Screw-like adapters on the end of each lumen that allow caps, syringes and intravenous tubing to be connected to them
- Hickman lines have plastic clamps on each lumen to close the catheter when it is not in use, or when disconnecting a cap, syringe or intravenous tubing.

CVCs are recommended for short-term use, due to the potential risk of infection (Loveday *et al.* 2014), and all devices should be removed as soon as they are no longer required.

How are CVCs inserted?

CVCs can be inserted in the operating theatre, or at the bedside under sterile conditions (depending on the type of catheter used).

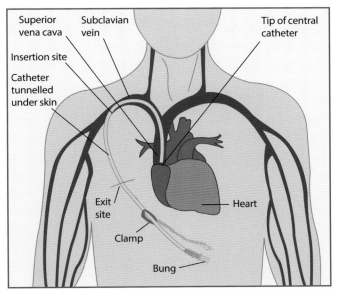

Figure 3.1 Central venous catheter placement

A tunnelled catheter is surgically inserted into a vein in the neck or chest and passed under the skin. One end of the catheter remains outside the skin. Medicines can be given through an opening at this end of the catheter. Passing the catheter under the skin helps keep it in place better, lets the patient move around more easily, and makes it less visible.

An alternative to this is an implanted port. An implanted port is similar to a tunnelled catheter, but the device is left entirely under the skin. It is normally placed below the clavicle into the right atrium of the heart, and is used for occasional or intermittent intravenous access. Medication is injected through the skin and into the catheter channel. An implanted port is less obvious than a tunnelled catheter, making it less visible and more acceptable to the patient.

How should healthcare professionals care for CVCs safely and effectively?

Following insertion, the catheter site needs to be regularly checked for signs of bleeding, redness, warmth or discharge. The signs of catheter-related problems and infection are similar for all types of CVCs.

The healthcare professional needs to monitor the patient for the following signs and symptoms:

● Redness, tenderness, warmth or odour around the catheter site

● Temperature of above 38° (or chills)

● Swelling of the face, neck, chest or arm on the side where the catheter is inserted

● Leakage of blood or fluid at the catheter site or the cap

● Inability to flush the catheter, or resistance when flushing the catheter

● Displacement (or lengthening) of the catheter.

Your local healthcare provider will have clinical guidelines for CVC care, and it is essential to familiarise yourself with them. These guidelines will vary, depending on where the CVC is being managed – in a hospital setting or in the patient's home. Many patients at home will be taught to manage the care of their catheter themselves, with support from their local community nursing team.

Remember: you must always wash your hands with liquid soap and water, rinse them well and then dry them thoroughly. You must also wear personal protective equipment before and after touching the CVC (Loveday *et al.* 2014). To prevent infection, anything that touches the exit site or goes into the CVC must be sterile. An aseptic non-touch technique (ANTT) must be followed at all times when handling the CVC.

ANTT is a technique that was originally developed by Rowley (2001); it maintains asepsis and is non-touch in nature. ANTT is supported by evidence, highlights the key components involved in maintaining asepsis and aims to standardise practice.

The underlying principles of ANTT are:

● Always wash hands effectively

● Never contaminate key parts

● Touch non-key parts with confidence

● Take appropriate precautions against infection.

ANTT should be used for both central and peripheral line care, as Rowley (2001) argues that it can be counterproductive to promote two different techniques.

The following guidelines are useful in preventing infection:

● Only use sterile supplies – discard any products in opened or damaged packaging

● Do not touch the end of the CVC when the cap has been removed

● If the CVC has a clamp, keep it clamped when not in use

- Remember to wash your hands thoroughly before and after working with the CVC
- Apply strict ANTT principles as part of your CVC care
- Always wear personal protective equipment – sterile gloves and an apron must be worn as a minimum requirement.

The CVC will normally be secured in place with a transparent dressing, unless it is an implanted port in which case a dressing will not be required. A transparent dressing is normally changed every 7 days (or more frequently if it becomes loose, damaged or soiled).

All dressing changes need to be undertaken using a strict aseptic technique to avoid the possibility of infection. Loveday et al. (2014) recommend daily cleansing with 2% chlorhexidine gluconate in 70% isopropyl alcohol in adult patients with a CVC, as a strategy to reduce infection. Iodine in alcohol can be used as an alternative for patients with sensitivity to chlorhexidine (Loveday et al. 2014).

What are the advantages and disadvantages of using PVADs?

Administration of IV therapy using a peripheral venous access device (PVAD) is simpler and cheaper and insertion is less traumatic for the patient, compared to inserting a CVC.

The disadvantages of using a PVAD include the fact that they are only suitable for a shorter period of use, they have a tendency to block more easily, and they have an increased risk of complications. (Complications associated with IV therapy will be discussed further in Chapter 8.)

Site selection for PVADs

The median, cephalic or basilic veins of the lower arm are most commonly used for peripheral access because they are located just beneath the skin (Richardson 2008). The cephalic vein is naturally very large, which makes it an excellent vessel for cannulation. The cephalic vein runs up the lateral side of the arm, from the hand to the forearm, up to the shoulder (humerus). Its position, by the radius in the forearm, also provides a natural splint. The basilic vein is similar to the cephalic vein, in that it is a large vessel which appears prominent, and is lightly supported by the ulna in the forearm. However, the basilic vein can 'roll' during insertion of the device, making insertion problematic (McCall & Tankersley 2008).

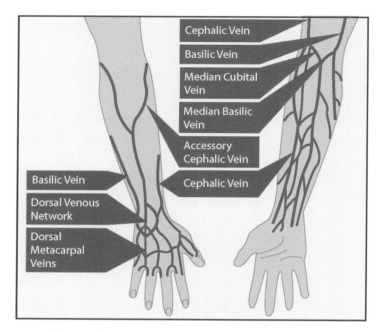

Cephalic Vein

Basilic Vein

Median Cubital Vein

Median Basilic Vein

Accessory Cephalic Vein

Basilic Vein

Cephalic Vein

Dorsal Venous Network

Dorsal Metacarpal Veins

Figure 3.2 The veins of the arm and the hand

An alternative to using the veins in the lower arm is to cannulate in the metacarpal veins (the veins located on the back of the hand). The metacarpal bones in the hand can assist in securing the device in position (Scales 2008) by acting as a splint. The disadvantage of metacarpal veins is that they are often smaller in diameter than those in the lower arm, and at times small veins are difficult to stabilise when inserting a PVAD. This is a particular problem with elderly or frail patients or for individuals with fragile veins.

If a suitable site for IV access cannot be found in either the upper limbs or the hands, it may be necessary to use the superficial veins of the lower limb, specifically the dorsum of the foot or the saphenous vein of the ankle. The Royal College of Nursing (RCN 2010) do not advocate the routine use of foot veins or veins in the lower limb due to the increased risk of complications, particularly thrombophlebitis and pulmonary embolism (Weinstein & Hagle 2014). Patients with diabetes must not have an IV access device placed in their foot (RCN 2010).

Site selection for a PVAD should be determined in line with the manufacturer's guide for insertion (Hamilton 2000). A thorough holistic assessment of the patient is essential, including assessment of the patient's condition, age and diagnosis (RCN 2010). An IV device can be intrusive and uncomfortable and may potentially impair limb extension and flexion, so effective patient assessment is needed to promote patient comfort, and to reduce any potential complications associated with insertion.

According to McCallum and Higgins (2012), the following points need to be considered when inserting a PVAD:

- The general condition of the patient's veins
- The need to avoid points of flexion (around joints)
- The medication to be administered
- How quickly the medication will be administered
- The patient's previous infusion device history
- The duration of the intended IV therapy
- The size of the PVAD compared with the size of the vein.

PVAD size selection

There are a range of different PVAD sizes (known as gauges) available. The smallest possible should be inserted to prevent damage to the vein, and allow administered medicines or therapies to 'mix' with the blood (Hadaway & Millam 2005). A smaller device will also be less uncomfortable for the patient, which is an equally important consideration.

Table 3.1 PVAD gauge sizes

Gauge size	General manufacturer colour	Approximate flow rate	Common uses
22g	Blue	40mL/min	• Small, fragile veins • Short-term access
20g	Pink	65mL/min	• Routine infusions • Post-operatively • Bolus drug administration
18g	Green	100mL/min	• Rapid infusions • Surgical and trauma patients
16g	Grey	210mL/min	• Major trauma or surgery • Massive fluid replacement
14g	Orange	270mL/min	• Emergency situations

Note: The manufacturer colour may vary from one country to another.

The overall size of the PVAD is determined by four factors – the needle gauge, the external diameter, the length and the flow rate in mL/min. The PVAD size is easily identifiable as injection port caps or chambers of the device are colour coded by manufacturers for easy recognition.

The healthcare practitioner needs to remember that as the device gauge number increases, the device bore gets smaller. For example, a blue PVAD has a 22g gauge, an external diameter of 0.8mm and a length of 25mm. In comparison, an orange device has a 14g gauge, with an external diameter of 2.1mm and a length of 45mm.

How should healthcare professionals care for PVADs safely and effectively?

Care must always be performed using an aseptic non-touch technique (ANTT) (Dougherty & Watson 2008). The Department of Health (2011) recommend that intravenous PVADs are checked twice daily as a minimum requirement. Of course, you should also familiarise yourself with your own healthcare provider's organisational policy or procedure for device care. The RCN (2010) recommend that the site is assessed when administering IV medication, changing bags of IV fluid or monitoring drip flow rates.

As a minimum standard for providing PVAD care, the healthcare practitioner needs to observe the device and surrounding area, as well as evaluating the integrity of the device and the security of any connections. Observation and monitoring of the site is essential to ensure that potential complications (such as phlebitis) are reduced, and that any significant change regarding the device (or the skin surrounding the device) is reported and responded to appropriately.

The site must be covered with a transparent dressing to ensure that it is visible at all times. The dressing should be made of sterile, occlusive and semi-permeable polyurethane (Loveday et al. 2014); non-sterile tape should not be used (McCallum 2012). A transparent dressing is permeable to water vapour and oxygen, but impermeable to micro-organisms (Loveday et al. 2014).

The dressing applied to the device site is the first line of defence against infection, and must always be kept secure, clean and dry. Correct application of the dressing will keep the IV device secure, by minimising movement in the lumen of the vein, and will reduce the risk of mechanical phlebitis (Higginson 2011). If the dressing becomes damp or loose, or there is blood or fluid leakage, it must be removed and changed immediately.

Dressings should also be changed according to the manufacturer's instructions. Dougherty and Watson (2008) point out that the dressing must not be secured with a bandage, as this causes moisture retention. Bandaging the area also obstructs visibility, making it impossible to observe the insertion site.

The High Impact Intervention Peripheral Intravenous Care bundle (DH 2011) advocates that PVAD ports should be cleaned with 2% chlorhexidine gluconate in 70% isopropyl alcohol prior to administration of medication (DH 2011), unless the patient is sensitive to chlorhexidine. The port of the device must be allowed to dry thoroughly prior to any administration. Loveday *et al.* (2014) recommend that the access port should be cleaned for a minimum of 15 seconds, and allowed to dry before accessing the system.

It is important that the PVAD is flushed with 5mL sodium chloride 0.9% at established intervals (e.g. before and after each administration of medicine, or every 24 hours if the device is not in use). The device must be flushed according to the healthcare provider's policy and clinical procedures, using an aseptic non-touch technique (ANTT), and the practitioner must ensure that the PVAD is patent before using it. The need for a PVAD should be reviewed on a daily basis; and it should be removed as soon as it is no longer required (DH 2011, Loveday *et al.* 2014).

Table 3.2 Minimum standards in PVAD care

What to do	Why it's done
Inspect the device at least twice a day (DH 2011), or more frequently if the patient's clinical condition dictates.	• To ensure the device is positioned correctly • To observe for potential complications with the device
Flush with sodium chloride 0.9% using a 10mL syringe at established intervals, e.g. before and after each use of the device, or every 24 hours if the device is not in use, using an aseptic non-touch technique (ANTT).	• To maintain patency of the device
Adopt an ANTT when handling the PVAD/infusion sets, and avoid any 'break' in the infusion system. A closed system should be used to minimise the risk of infection.	• To avoid potential contamination entering the circulatory system through infection or a 'break'
Secure the device with a transparent, semi-occlusive dressing. Do not replace this unless it gets damp, damaged or soiled.	• To allow visual inspection of the device site • To reduce the risk of dislodgement or mechanical complications

Summary

This chapter has focused on the different types of PVADs that are used to administer IV fluids and/or medication. CVCs and PVADs have been broadly described, highlighting their respective advantages and modes of use, and identifying how best to care for and manage these devices. Ensure that you read and familiarise yourself with your local healthcare policy and guidelines so that you can meet the relevant standards for safe and effective practice within your specific clinical area.

Chapter 4

Calculating medication doses

Learning outcomes

At the end of this chapter, the practitioner will be able to:

- **Understand the importance of calculating medication doses accurately**
- **Understand the principles that underpin safe, accurate medicine calculation**
- **Demonstrate competency when calculating medication doses.**

Introduction

The National Patient Safety Agency (NPSA) reported a total of nearly 73,000 medication incidents in 2007 (NPSA 2009). While most of these incidents resulted in little or no harm to patients, the NPSA (2009) found that 41% resulted in serious harm or death and these were caused during the medication administration stage. In total, 5% of the incidents were directly attributable to the wrong dose of medication being administered (NPSA 2009).

Medication administration is a task that a healthcare practitioner performs on a daily basis, so it is vital to be able to calculate medication doses correctly. The healthcare practitioner needs to understand what they are doing, and be familiar with some of the commonly used dosage formulas. This knowledge will help the practitioner maintain safe practice with medicines administration.

Many of the errors reported by the National Patient Safety Agency (2009) could have been avoided if the calculation had been checked, and checked again. More often than not, it is human error that leads to mistakes being made.

What are the main points to remember when calculating medication?

Points for your practice

- Is the amount correct? Often it is not the number that is wrong, but the amount given (O'Brien et al. 2011).
- Ask yourself, is this a sensible answer?
- Have you used the correct dose (e.g. milligrams, not micrograms)?

Points for your practice

Remember, the weight of a medicine (using tablets or capsules) is usually measured in grams, milligrams or micrograms:

1000 MICROgrams make a MILLIgram (mg)

1000 MILLIgrams (mg) make a GRAM (g)

1000 GRAMs (g) make up a KILOgram (Kg) (the weight of a bag of sugar).

The British National Formulary (BNF) recommends that micrograms are written in full, rather than using the abbreviation mcg. This is to avoid confusion, and potential accidental medication overdose.

The 'conversion' factor using these types of weights is 1000. Look at the medication that you are preparing to administer and check how it is measured. If a medication is to be dissolved or suspended in a liquid, the liquid format is measured in LITRES (L) and MILLIlitres (mL). Here, the conversion factor of liquid is also 1000. You will need to calculate how much liquid to administer to your patient. Some medicines state that the medication needs to be prepared using a weight in a specific volume of fluid (e.g. 1mg per mL). This means that 1 MILLIgram (mg) of medication will be delivered per MILLIlitre (mL) of fluid administered, if it is prepared correctly.

Non-liquid forms of medication

Medications are manufactured in many different forms, such as liquid, tablets and powders. As this is a book about the administration of intravenous (IV) therapy, the examples provided will relate to liquid, in order to calculate doses that are appropriate for this route.

As a reminder, for medicines that are to be administered in a solid form (such as tablets or capsules), the basic formula for calculation is:

$$\frac{\text{What you want}}{\text{What you've got}} \quad or \quad \frac{\text{Prescribed dose}}{\text{Stock dosage (what's in the bottle)}}$$

For instance, paracetamol is dispensed as 500mg tablets. If a patient is prescribed 1 gram, the formula would be applied as:

$$\frac{\text{What you want}}{\text{What you've got}} \quad or \quad \frac{\text{Prescribed dose is 1 gram}}{\text{Stock dosage is 500mg}}$$

Medications in liquid form

Medications are often measured in grams. However, for IV administration, they need to be dissolved in a liquid or suspension format. Therefore, you need to calculate what amount of liquid to administer.

When calculating the quantity of medicine needed in a liquid form, the following formula can be used:

$$\frac{\text{What you want} \quad x \quad \text{the volume it is in}}{\text{What you've got}}$$

or

$$\frac{\text{Prescribed dose} \quad x \quad \text{volume of stock dosage}}{\text{Stock dosage (what's in the bottle)}}$$

Example 4.1

Here is an example to help you apply the formula:

A patient is prescribed 80mg of Drug A. The label on the medicine says there are 40mg in 2mL. How many mL do you think you need to administer?

First set the problem out, using the formula above:

Want: **80mg** (what you want)

Got: **40mg** (what you have got)

In: **2mL** (the volume it's in)

Applying the formula, your calculation will be:

$$\frac{80 \times 2}{40}$$

Your answer will be:

4mL

Activity 4.1

Think about some of the common medications that are used in your clinical area. How are these prepared and administered? Work out the calculations for the common doses that are used.

When you have worked out each calculation, check that it makes sense! Always stop and think – does it look as if there are too many tablets or too large a volume of liquid? Equally, is there a very small amount? Or do you need to split tablets? Always check your calculation again, and use a second checker if something does not look quite right.

Some medications are prescribed based on body weight. These medications are always calculated according to the patient's weight in kilograms (kg). This means that your prescription will be prescribed as milligrams (mg) per kg, micrograms per kg, etc. To calculate the correct dose, you will need to multiply the prescribed dose by the patient's weight in kilograms.

Example 4.2

A paediatric patient is prescribed dexamethasone 150 micrograms/kg. The patient weighs 8kg.

This means that the calculation is:

150 micrograms x 8 = 1200 micrograms *or* 1.2 milligrams (mg)

Calculating IV fluids

There are three stages to working out the rate at which IV fluids need to be administered. (A rate is known as an amount per unit of time.)

1. How many millilitres per hour need to be given?

2. How many millilitres per minute need to be given?

3. How many drops per minute need to be given?

In order to administer an IV infusion, you will need the correct administration set (often called a giving set). A clear fluid administration set delivers 20 drops of fluid per mL. The clear chamber in the middle of the administration set is used to count the drip rate (i.e. how many drops drip through the chamber per minute). Fluids will need to be administered at the prescribed rate, as detailed on the prescription.

If you are using an infusion device to deliver fluid, the device will have its own specific administration set devised by the manufacturer. Again, this administration set will deliver 20 drops of fluid per mL.

Blood, blood products or plasma expanding agents are typically administered using a specific administration set. These administration sets have filters, and deliver 15 drops of fluid per mL (Boyd 2013). This is because the fluid administered has a more viscous (thicker) consistency. Care of infusion lines and infusion devices will be discussed in Chapter 6.

Points for your practice

Remember the drops per mL will vary with the type of administration set used – and this will affect your calculation!

To calculate an infusion rate in drops per minute:

$$\text{Drops rate per minute} = \frac{\text{Volume in mL}}{\text{Time in hours}} \times \frac{\text{Drops per mL}}{60}$$

Example 4.3

1000mL sodium chloride 0.9% is prescribed to be administered over 8 hours. The administration set delivers 20 drops per mL. To calculate the drops per minute, the following formula would be applied:

Volume in mL = 1000 (as you have a 1000mL bag of fluid)

Time in hours = 8 (as it is to be administered over 8 hours)

Drops per mL = 20 (as your infusion set delivers 20 drops per mL)

This means that the calculation is:

$$\text{Drops rate per minute} = \frac{1000}{8} \times \frac{20}{60}$$

The answer is:

41.7 drops per minute.

As we cannot administer 0.7 of a drop, we round this up to a whole number, which equals 42 drops per minute.

Activity 4.2

Practise the following calculations to work out the drops per minute:

1. 500mL of 5% dextrose is prescribed to be administered over 4 hours. The administration set delivers 20 drops per mL.

2. 500mL of whole blood is prescribed to be administered over 4 hours. The administration set delivers 15 drops per mL.

3. 1000mL of Hartmann's solution is prescribed to be administered over 6 hours. The administration set delivers 20 drops per mL.

The answers to this activity are in Appendix 4.

Working out how long an infusion will last when infused at a specific rate

Sometimes you might need to work out how long an infusion will last. This is relevant if you are required to administer an infusion at a specific rate.

To calculate how long an infusion will last when infused at a specific rate, use the following formula:

$$\text{Time fluid will last (in hours)} = \frac{\text{Volume in mL}}{\text{Rate of drops per min}} \times \frac{\text{Drops per mL}}{60}$$

Example 4.4

500mL of whole blood is to be transfused at 25 drops per minute. The administration set delivers at 15 drops per mL. How long will the blood last?

Volume in mL = 500mL (as you have a 500mL bag of fluid)

Drops per mL = 15 (as your infusion set delivers 15 drops per mL)

Drops per minute = 25 (as your infusion is set to deliver 25 drops per minute)

This means that the calculation is:

$$\text{Time infusion will last (in hours)} = \frac{500}{25} \times \frac{15}{60}$$

The answer is:

5 hours

Activity 4.3

Practise the following calculations to work out how long each infusion will last:

1. 500mL of 5% dextrose is prescribed to be administered at 20 drops per minute. The administration set delivers 20 drops per mL.

2. 500mL of whole blood is prescribed to be administered at 40 drops per minute. The administration set delivers 15 drops per mL.

3. 100mL of Hartmann's solution is prescribed to be administered at 10 drops per minute. The administration set delivers 20 drops per mL.

The answers to this activity are in Appendix 4.

Chapter 5

How drugs work – an introduction to pharmacokinetics and pharmacodynamics

Learning outcomes

At the end of this chapter, the practitioner will be able to:

- **Demonstrate the principles of safe medication administration**
- **Understand what pharmacodynamics means**
- **Understand the general principles of pharmacokinetics**
- **Understand what is meant by adverse drug reactions and medication interactions.**

Introduction

Prior to the administration of medication by any route (not just intravenous), the healthcare practitioner must demonstrate an adequate level of knowledge of:

- Pharmacokinetics, i.e. the way medication is absorbed, distributed, metabolised and eliminated
- Key issues such as patient consent, professional accountability, negligence, and vicarious liability (NMC 2008)
- The local healthcare provider's policy on medicines management
- How to calculate drug dosages effectively.

The principles of safe medication administration

The healthcare practitioner must equally demonstrate safe, evidence-based practice, and have due regard for their level of competence and patient safety (Endacott, Jevon & Cooper 2009). To ensure safe administration of medication, it is very helpful to memorise the '5 Rs' checklist (Clayton 1987):

● Right patient
● Right drug
● Right route
● Right dose
● Right time.

The healthcare practitioner must also be able to demonstrate adequate knowledge of the specific medication that is being administered. This includes:

● Action and indications for the medicine being used
● Side effects
● Any contra-indications
● Potential medication interactions
● Need for patient monitoring (pre-dose, during administration and post-dose)
● Normal therapeutic dose and range of doses
● Storage, stability, usability (or potential for contamination) and expiry date
● Sources of advice and support (e.g. local clinical guidelines, pharmacist, etc.)
● Any legislation relating to the type of medicine being administered.

Activity 5.1

Find and read the following pieces of legislation on http://www.legislation.gov. uk/. Then consider how each one addresses the administration of medication:
• **The Medicines Act (1968)**
• **The Misuse of Drugs Act (1971)**
• **Health Act (2006)**
• **Controlled Drugs (Supervision of Management and Use) Regulations (2013)**

Understanding pharmacodynamics

As a healthcare practitioner, it is important to have a good working knowledge of how medicines work, and how an individual's body can affect a medication that is administered. Pharmacodynamics focuses on 'what the medication does to the body'. In most cases, pharmacodynamics is the study of a medication's interaction with an intended receptor (or target within the body) that binds the medication given to an individual's physiological system.

For most medicines to work, they must target a receptor in the body, or a particular micro-organism (such as a bacterial infection). A receptor is a specific type of protein that sticks out from a cell's body. The medication includes a different protein, called a ligand, which can connect with that particular receptor. The two proteins snap together, like pieces in a jigsaw puzzle, and the binding acts like a trigger, setting a course of chemical reactions in motion, and thus beginning the process of combating a disease.

Knowing which sort of ligand to attach to a medicine is an important part of pharmacodynamics. One of the most significant areas of pharmacodynamics is ensuring that medicines are efficient across a wide range of ages and stages of disease. Medicines need receptors to bind to. Medications may therefore need to be created with multiple ligands, which can bind to multiple receptors to cover a broad age range.

Another facet of pharmacodynamics concerns the effects that a medication might have in the body, once it has bound to its intended receptor. Medicines are supposed to change what is happening in the body. For instance, they can alter how a virus is replicating; they can inhibit tumour growth or strengthen the immune system. In the early stages of medication development, pharmacodynamics is used to study the unintended consequences of medicine binding. These side effects might include causing damage to the body's cells, inducing cell mutation leading to cancerous growths, or (in a worst-case scenario) increasing a disease's potency.

All our body systems are mediated by control systems, which depend upon genetic make-up, DNA and enzyme production. When an individual receives a medicine, it interferes with these systems, and the interaction of the medication within our body's cells produces a biochemical or physiological change. To work effectively, the medication given must reach the target cell in the body in either a specific or non-specific way.

Medications work in one of the following ways:

- Replacing a deficiency to provide a normal physiological response (e.g. insulin is administered for diabetes mellitus)
- Affecting cell growth and division (e.g. chemotherapy is used to target cancer cells)

- Interfering with micro-organisms (germs) that invade the body – either by killing germs directly or by preventing them from multiplying and growing
- Changing the way cells work in the body. Most common chronic diseases (such as hypertension, arthritis, heart disease, and some types of mental illness) are caused by cells functioning abnormally. These abnormalities may be caused by cell ageing, genetics and lifestyle issues (such as smoking, lack of exercise, poor eating habits, and environmental stress and pollution). Medications work to target these cell abnormalities.

Understanding pharmacokinetics

Pharmacokinetics is essentially the reverse of pharmacodynamics. Pharmacokinetics is the study of what the body does to a drug (medicine). In simple terms this is the study of drug transport through the body (pharma = drug, kinetics = movement) (Endacott, Jevon & Cooper 2009). In order to be effective, the medication needs to be available at the right site, in the right concentration and at the right time.

Medication also needs to be administered using a suitable route, absorbed through the skin, bronchi or gastro-intestinal tract, and distributed to the site of action (generally through the circulation). For intravenous (IV) therapy, the absorption phase of pharmacokinetics is bypassed, as the medicine is being administered directly into the circulatory system, and it is ready to be distributed appropriately. Following distribution, the medication is broken down (metabolised), and finally excreted (or removed) from the body.

Absorption

Absorption is the movement of the medicine from the administration site into the circulatory system. Essentially, absorption brings the medicine into the bloodstream. The amount of the medicine absorbed and the rate of absorption can vary, depending on certain factors:

- The nature of the dosage form (e.g. tablet or capsule)
- Whether or not food is present in the stomach
- The composition of the gastric/intestinal PH
- Whether or not other drugs are being administered at the same time
- The mesenteric blood flow.

Bioavailability

Bioavailability is the term used to identify the proportion of the administered medication that reaches the circulatory system. Bioavailability refers to the amount of the medication that is available to be distributed to the intended site of action. Drugs administered using an IV route are considered to have 100 per cent bioavailability (Boyd 2013).

Distribution

When a medication enters the circulatory system, it is diluted and transported around the body. This is known as the distribution phase. Movement from blood to the tissues can be influenced by numerous factors. Plasma protein can bind to medication, meaning that only the unbound portion is free to move from the bloodstream into the tissues, where it has a pharmacological effect. The blood-brain barrier within the nervous system is highly selective for lipid-soluble (fat-soluble) medicines. For example, penicillin diffuses well within body tissues, but does not penetrate well into the cerebrospinal fluid (Boyd 2013). The placenta provides a barrier between the mother and foetus during pregnancy. Some medicines cross the placenta easily (e.g. morphine), whereas others do not.

Metabolism

Metabolism modifies or alters the chemical composition of the medicine, ready for the final phase, excretion. The main site of metabolism is the liver, but other organs or tissues may metabolise medicines, such as the lungs, kidneys, blood and intestine. Not all medications are metabolised – digoxin, for example, is excreted unchanged.

Most medication interactions occur during the metabolism phase; and this can cause unwanted side effects, or increase the action of a medicine. Some medication interactions can be particularly harmful to patients.

Activity 5.2

What factors do you think predispose some patient groups to medication interaction?

Medication interactions

There are many factors that can predispose an individual to medications potentially interacting:

- Age – as we get older, physiological changes occur that may affect the interaction of medicines. Our liver metabolism, kidney function and nerve transmission all decrease with age.
- Polypharmacy – the more medications an individual takes, the higher the risk of them interacting with each other, leading to unwanted effects.
- Genetic factors – our individual genetic make-up can increase or decrease enzyme activity.
- Hepatic or renal diseases – medicines that are metabolised in the liver and/or eliminated by the kidneys may be altered if these organs are not functioning correctly.

Another factor to consider is the consumption of certain types of food and drink when taking medicines. Food can influence the way a drug is metabolised; alcohol is the best-known example of this. Individuals who drink alcohol and take paracetamol regularly are at significant risk of developing liver damage.

Other common foodstuffs can that affect medications are grapefruit juice (affects Nifedipine and Midazolam), garlic (affects anti-coagulants) and chamomile (affects benzodiazepines and opioids). Always check the patient information leaflet for such interactions prior to administering medicines.

Excretion

The final phase of pharmacokinetics is excretion. Medicines are excreted by the kidney (with the exception of anaesthetic gases, which are excreted unchanged through the respiratory tract). The rate of excretion varies; some medicines are excreted quickly, whereas others may take days or even weeks. It is important to consider patients with predisposing medical conditions, as this may affect medication elimination rates – for example, patients with renal impairment may excrete medicines more slowly. If the dose is not reduced, the plasma levels of the drug will increase, potentially producing a poisonous (toxic) effect (Boyd 2013).

Understanding adverse reactions to medication

An individual can have many responses to the medicines they are given, ranging from an adverse reaction (an undesirable or unwanted response) to severe allergy or anaphylaxis. This happens when a severe immune response is mediated by the reaction to a medicine. An adverse reaction refers to the harm caused by a medication given at a normal dose and during normal use.

An adverse reaction may be produced by any medicine administered; no medicine is entirely free from causing side effects. These side effects may include unpleasant symptoms, such as nausea and vomiting, dizziness, gastro-intestinal disturbances, urticaria or pruritus. The British National Formulary (BNF) lists side effects in order of frequency, ranging from very common (more than 1 in 10), to less common (from 1 in 1000 to 1 in 100) and rare (fewer than 1 in 10,000).

Activity 5.3

Look up the common IV medications used in your clinical area. Read the patient information leaflet supplied with the medicine. What are the common adverse reactions?

In the United Kingdom, the Medicines and Healthcare Products Regulatory Agency (MHRA) studies adverse drug medication reactions by overseeing medicines that are taken by patients, and also the use of medical devices. If a healthcare practitioner suspects that a medication has caused an adverse reaction, they should report it.

It is often difficult to establish that it is definitely the medicine that has caused a side effect, but the standard reporting form, through the use of a 'yellow card', can be found in the British National Formulary (BNF). The yellow card and information for completion can be accessed on line at www.yellowcard.gov.uk. Once this information is reported, the MHRA can establish whether the medication risk is common or serious, and decide on a course of action. The MHRA will consider the potential risks associated with the side effects of the medicine, and the risk to the patient if the condition is not treated. Medicines are very rarely removed from the market.

Summary

This chapter has introduced the principles of safe administration of medication, and has identified and discussed how medicines work, their effects on the body and the potential for adverse reactions. You will need to study in detail each medication that you plan to administer to ensure that it is safe to do so, and that you have sufficient information and knowledge of that particular medicine.

Chapter 6

Safe administration of intravenous fluids and medicines

Learning outcomes

At the end of this chapter, the practitioner will be able to:

- **Understand the different methods of delivering intravenous fluids and/or medication**
- **Select the appropriate equipment needed to safely administer intravenous fluid**
- **Understand the step-by-step process in relation to the safe administration of intravenous fluid**
- **Select the appropriate equipment needed to prepare intravenous medication**
- **Understand the step-by-step process in relation to the safe administration of intravenous medication**
- **Demonstrate how to provide appropriate patient monitoring and aftercare.**

Introduction

It is important to follow your local healthcare provider's policy and clinical guidelines when administering intravenous (IV) fluid and/or medications. Some policies provide detailed information, and include step-by-step guidelines, as well as explaining why things are performed in a specific way. In order to administer IV therapy, it is likely that you will need to attend an additional training session and have a period of supervised practice with an appropriately qualified practitioner. Lastly, you will need to be assessed to ensure that you are competent to undertake the procedure.

Understanding different methods of delivery

The method used to deliver IV therapy depends upon numerous factors, such as the drug being used, the patient's condition and the desired effect of the drug. There are three main methods for delivering IV medication – through a continuous infusion, an intermittent infusion or a bolus method, which is sometimes referred to as an intermittent injection (Dougherty 2002).

Continuous infusion

IV fluid and/or medication can also be delivered in a larger volume of solution. This is known as a continuous infusion method (Boyd 2013). A continuous infusion is typically used to administer IV fluids, or when medication needs to be well diluted (Dougherty 2002). Alternatively, a continuous infusion method may be advocated when the plasma level of the medicine needs to be maintained, or when large volumes of fluid and electrolyte need to be replaced (Dougherty 2002).

An example of a continuous infusion is the administration of 1000mL sodium chloride 0.9%, used as maintenance fluid when the patient has restricted oral intake (e.g. when they are 'nil by mouth'). However, there are some disadvantages to using a continuous infusion method, such as the risk of fluid overload, or the incompatibility between the infusion and other IV drugs administered through the same peripheral access device (Weinstein & Hagle 2014).

Intermittent infusion

An intermittent infusion method is used when a medication is added to a small volume of fluid (between 50 and 250mL), and administered over a prescribed period of time, which can vary between 20 minutes and 2 hours (Dougherty 2002). The intermittent infusion method may be used for a specific one-off dose, or alternatively administered at repeated intervals within a 24-hour period (Weinstein & Hagle 2014). Between doses of the medication, the container and the administration set must be discontinued, removed and discarded.

An intermittent infusion method is used when the pharmacology (or make-up) of the medication dictates a specific dilution, or if the medication becomes unstable if delivered and administered in a more dilute volume of fluid. An intermittent infusion may be used, for instance, if the patient is on a restricted fluid intake. Intermittent infusion is also used to administer antibiotics. The disadvantages of this approach include the requirement to use additional equipment, and the risk that an increased concentration of the medication may cause venous irritation (Weinstein & Hagle 2014).

Bolus method

A bolus method (also known as a direct intermittent injection) is the administration of a small volume of medication being pushed into the peripheral vascular access device (PVAD) or central venous catheter (CVC), using a 'needle-free' device (in which the syringe can be twisted onto the cap of an access device to provide an administration route).

Medication must be administered slowly using this method, over a time period ranging from a few minutes to 30 minutes, depending upon the medicine (Dougherty 2002). This approach may be used when a rapid dose of the drug is needed (e.g. in an emergency situation) and an immediate response is required, or when the medication cannot be diluted for pharmacological or therapeutic reasons (Dougherty 2002). The main disadvantage of this method is that it can cause a rapid delivery of the medicine, potentially causing a toxic effect or an anaphylactic reaction.

A bolus method is additionally used to administer sodium chloride 0.9% flushes to keep the PVAD patent. When administering a flush, a 'push pause' method is advocated, meaning that you must stop and start the administration of the fluid (Boyd 2013). The 'push pause' method creates episodes of turbulence, which removes small particles of debris that can build up around the tip of the PVAD (Boyd 2013). Remember that all flushes must be prescribed (or form part of a patient group directive) prior to their administration.

Activity 6.1

Identify a commonly used IV medication that is used in your clinical area. Study the medication in detail – think about how it is mixed, what diluent is used, and the method of administration. Next, identify the side effects of the medication, and consider the effects it may have on the patient's vein. You may find it useful to create a 'drug diary' to list the common IV medications used within your clinical area.

Preparing the patient for administration of IV fluid or medication

Once a patient assessment has been undertaken, and the need for IV therapy has been determined, you need to prepare the patient fully by obtaining their consent and explaining the reason for the IV therapy. Patient education should also include the likely duration of the IV therapy and the possible side effects (Lavery & Ingram 2008). In addition, the patient's prescription chart and notes should be checked for any other medication that the patient is receiving, to eliminate any possible drug interactions, incompatibilities, known allergies or side effects (Lavery & Ingram 2008).

Points for your practice

Before administering any medication (Boyd 2013):

● Explain the steps in the procedure to the patient

● Use the '5 Rs' checklist to support your practice (see p. 32)

● Ensure you know the identity of the patient you are administering the medicine to

● Familiarise yourself with the medication and any contraindications.

Preparing equipment for administration of IV fluid or medication

Preparation of the equipment depends upon the chosen route of IV therapy (i.e. whether the therapy is to be given through a continuous, intermittent or bolus method).

The main points for good practice are as follows:

● Check that the patient has appropriate IV access, and that the access device is patent, prior to assembling your equipment or fluid/medication to be infused.

● Wash your hands as per aseptic non-touch technique (ANTT) national guidance.

● The PVAD must be flushed with 5mL sodium chloride 0.9% (using a 10mL syringe), using a 'push pause' technique (Boyd 2013).

● Check that the prescription is correct and valid, and that the dose required has not already been administered (NMC 2008).

- Always use single use equipment as appropriate (Medical Devices Agency 2000). Check that the equipment is in date, has been stored correctly and is not damaged, to ensure that the product is safe to use (Lavery & Ingram 2008).
- Assemble all equipment to reconstitute (draw up) the medication safely, so that there is no delay in administration.
- Assess the area for immediate risks, and ensure that it is safe and suitable for medication administration. The area should be clean with sufficient space, light and ventilation to allow the medication to be prepared safely.
- Check that you have appropriate equipment to deal with any spillages quickly and effectively.
- Always ensure that you wear personal protective equipment; gloves and an apron is a required minimum standard (Loveday et al. 2014). If there is a risk of splashing (e.g. when preparing and mixing medication), you should wear protective eye goggles.

Administering IV fluid via a continuous infusion (without adding a medicine)

Before administering any IV fluid, you will need to ensure that there is a valid prescription in place. A typical prescription will resemble the one shown in Figure 6.1 (below). Make sure that the prescription is accurate (e.g. check that the date, volume and fluid type are correct) and that the prescriber has signed and printed their name on the prescription. If you are in any doubt, or the prescription is incorrect, do NOT administer the IV fluid.

Date	Intravenous fluid	Volume	Duration	Additive	Prescriber's signature	Batch number	Nurse's signature	Time started	Time completed
A date	5% dextrose	1000mL	8 hours	None	A. Prescriber				

Figure 6.1 A typical prescription slip

In order to administer a continuous infusion of IV fluid, you will need the correct administration set (often called a giving set). A clear fluid administration set delivers 20 drops of fluid per mL. The clear chamber in the middle of the administration set is used to count the drip rate (i.e. how many drops drip through the chamber each minute). This type of administration set needs to be changed every 72 hours (Royal College of Nursing 2010). Fluids must be administered at the prescribed rate, as detailed on the prescription.

If you are using an infusion device to deliver fluid, the device will have its own specific administration set devised by the manufacturer. Again, this administration set will deliver 20 drops of fluid per mL, and will require changing every 72 hours (Royal College of Nursing 2010). It is good practice to label the line with the date and time of commencement, so that other practitioners are aware of when to change infusion lines.

Blood and blood products are typically administered over a 3- to 4-hour period, using a specific blood administration set. Blood administration sets have filters, and deliver 15 drops of fluid per mL (Boyd 2013). The administration set will require changing every 12 hours.

Points for your practice

You will need to calculate the flow rate of an infusion in drops per minute, using the following formula:

$$\text{Flow rate (drops/min)} = \frac{\text{volume of a solution (mL)} \times \text{number of drops per mL}}{\text{Duration of infusion (in minutes)}}$$

Example 6.1

If you wanted to administer 100mL sodium chloride 0.9% over 30 minutes, using a standard giving set, the calculation would be as follows:

Volume of solution = 100mL

Number of drops per mL = 20 (as you are using a standard IV infusion giving set)

Duration of infusion = 30 minutes

$$\frac{100 \text{ (mL)} \times 20 \text{ (drops)}}{30 \text{ (minutes)}} = 66.6 \text{ drops per minute}$$

Now practise some infusion calculations in Activity 6.2.

Activity 6.2

If I litre (IL) 5% glucose is prescribed and to be administered over 8 hours, using a standard giving set delivering 20 drops per mL, what would the infusion rate be in drops per minute?

If 500mL sodium chloride is prescribed and to be administered over 2 hours, using a standard giving set delivering 20 drops per mL, what would the infusion rate be in drops per minute?

If I litre (IL) 5% glucose is prescribed and to be administered over 6 hours, using a standard giving set delivering 20 drops per mL, what would the infusion rate be in drops per minute?

(The answers to this activity are in Appendix 4.)

Once you have checked the prescription and determined that it is accurate, gather the fluid and equipment, calculate the flow rate according to the above formula, and ask a second checker to check the fluid and the calculation with you against the patient's prescription chart. You should go to the patient together to check the fluid against the prescription, and against the correct patient.

Flush the PVAD with 5mL sodium chloride 0.9% (using a 10mL syringe), and set up the fluid ready for administration. Once you have commenced the IV infusion, check the flow rate, dispose of your equipment, and then immediately sign and date the prescription chart, as well as documenting what time the infusion commenced. When the infusion is complete, you can document the completion time. Many healthcare providers require a second checker's signature on the prescription chart (where appropriate) in addition to the signature of the person administering the fluid.

When a patient has an IV infusion running, they will also need their fluid balance to be recorded. The core principle of fluid balance is that the amount of water lost from the body must equal the amount of water taken in. For example, in human homeostasis, the output must equal the input. It is important that a fluid balance chart is started, so that all fluid input (oral drinks, IV fluids, IV medications, etc.) and all fluid output (urine, vomit, wound drains, etc.) can be documented accurately. This will allow you to work out the patient's daily fluid balance (or fluid input minus output).

Table 6.1 Key stages in preparing and administering IV fluid using a continuous infusion method, without adding a medication (additive)

What is done	Why it is done
1. Collect all the equipment required (prescribed fluid, suitable IV administration set; 5mL sodium chloride 0.9% flush, prepared in a 10mL syringe). Sterile pack containing waste bag and gauze swabs; Wound care pack; Sodium chloride; Apron Gloves; Transparent dressing; Swab; 1000mL infusion bag; 23-gauge needle; 10mL syringe; 0.9% sodium chloride; Administration set; Alternatively, 10mL syringe pre-filled with 0.9% sodium chloride	To ensure that the healthcare practitioner has everything they need, and the procedure can be carried out quickly and effectively. ◄ *Figure 6.2 Gather all the equipment needed*
2. Wash your hands with soap and water, and apply the ANTT principles.	To avoid contamination from the healthcare practitioner.
3. Make sure that your second checker is with you to check the fluid against the prescription, and that you have identified the correct patient.	To ensure that you have the correct patient (NPSA 2006).
4. Obtain consent from the patient.	To ensure that the patient understands and agrees that they are willing to undergo the procedure.
5. Inspect the fluid packaging; confirm that it is the correct fluid for administration, the fluid is clear, the bag is not leaking, and that it is in date. Open the packaging and place the bag on a flat sterile surface, preferably in a tray to avoid spillages. *(NB: Sterile packaging should not be damaged or wet.)* If any problems are identified, discard the fluid and start again.	To avoid any risk of cross-contamination.

6. Ensure that you have the correct giving set for the administration of the fluid.	To reduce potential waste.
7. Open the packaging for the IV giving set, open it out, but do not let the ends touch anything, as you will need to protect the key parts. Close the roller clamp (flow regulator). 	To avoid contamination and the potential for infection. ◀ *Figure 6.3 Open the packaging* ◀ *Figure 6.4 Close the roller clamp*
8. Remove the port from the bag of IV fluid, and the protective cap from the spike of the administration set.	To prepare the equipment to be assembled.

9. **Insert the spike of the administration set into the port of the fluid bag. Push and twist slightly to insert it into position. Be careful not to puncture the bag, or yourself. Make sure that you insert the spike fully into the infusion bag. 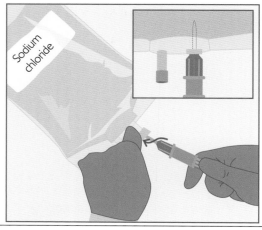	To avoid puncturing the bag and subsequently contaminating the fluid. ◄ *Figure 6.5 Insert the spike*
10. Hold the infusion bag higher than the drip chamber on the administration set. Squeeze the drip chamber to start the flow of fluid. (Fill the drip chamber until it is one-third full.)	To encourage filling of the administration set.
11. Open the flow regulator and allow the fluid to flush all air from the tubing, to the end of the administration set. Take care not to touch the tip of the administration set, or allow it to become contaminated. 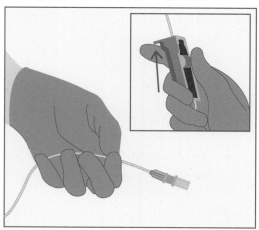	To reduce the risk of air being trapped in the line. ◄ *Figure 6.6 Prime the infusion line*

The primed set is ready to be connected to the patient. Set up your infusion pump (if this is the method you are using) or calculate the flow rate required for gravity-fed infusions.	
12. If the PVAD is not in use, clean the port with 2% chlorhexidine gluconate in 70% isopropyl alcohol (DH 2011) and allow to dry. Flush with 5mL sodium chloride 0.9% (using a 10mL syringe). Check that the PVAD is patent before you connect the infusion to the patient. 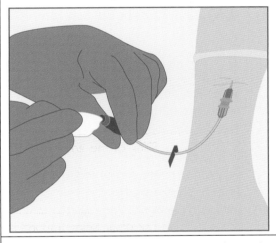	To ensure that the PVAD is clean and patent before it is used. ◀ *Figure 6.7 Clean the injection cap*
13. Connect the end of the tubing to the patient, and commence the infusion at the required rate. 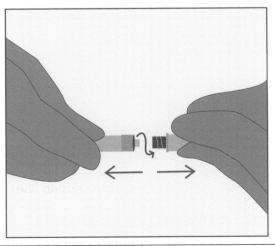	To administer the infusion at a safe rate. ◀ *Figure 6.8 Connect the tubing to the patient*

Check the flow rate.	
	◀ Figure 6.9 Check the flow rate
14. Remove personal protective equipment. Wash hands, dispose of equipment according to your local healthcare provider's policy.	To reduce the risk of cross contamination, and to ensure that correct disposal methods are adhered to.
15. Sign and document on the patient's prescription chart. Label the infusion set.	To document the time and date when the infusion commenced, and to identify when to change the infusion line; to adhere to the NMC Code (2015).
16. Commence a fluid balance chart, documenting the name of the fluid, and the volume that has been commenced.	To keep an accurate record of the patient's fluid balance.

Once the infusion has completed, you will need to stop the infusion and disconnect the infusion set. To do this, you will need to:

● Clamp the infusion set tubing. Switch off the infusion pump and remove the infusion giving set from the pump (if you are using one).

● Wash your hands with soap and water, and put on apron and gloves as a minimum standard for using personal protective equipment

● Using an aseptic non-touch technique, disconnect the infusion set from the PVAD or CVC site. Apply a new sterile cover (or bung).

● The PVAD site should be flushed with 5mL sodium chloride 0.9% (prepared in a 10mL syringe) to ensure that the device remains patent.

- Check the access site, and document accordingly. Take appropriate action if any complications are identified (see Chapter 7 for additional information on risk, complications and adverse reactions).
- Dispose of your equipment according to your local healthcare provider's policy, in a clinical waste bag and sharps container (where appropriate).

Preparing injectable intravenous medicines

If you are preparing an injectable medicine for intravenous administration, you will need to ensure that it is prepared and administered according to your local healthcare provider's policy and guidelines. There are many risks to both patients and practitioners when prescribing, preparing and administering injectable medicines.

The most common risks associated with injectable medicines have been identified by the National Patient Safety Agency (NPSA 2007). These include:

- A lack of information available to healthcare practitioners at the point of use.
- Incomplete prescriptions, which do not include important information (such as the diluent), the final volume of medication to be administered, or the intended rate of administration. There are also risks linked to the overuse of abbreviations on prescriptions.
- Supply and use of injectable medicines that may require complex calculation, dilution and handling procedures, as opposed to ready-to-use products.
- Calculation errors made during the prescription, preparation, administration of the medicine, leading to administration of the wrong dose and/or at the wrong concentration or rate.
- Unsafe handling or poor aseptic (non-touch) technique leading to contamination of the injection, and harm to the patient.
- Variable levels of knowledge, training and competence among healthcare practitioners.

When preparing an injectable medicine, you will find that it is manufactured in several different formulations; this is due to the stability of the medication itself. Formulations are categorised into:

- Aqueous solutions – medicines that are stable and ready to use (e.g. Heparin).
- Powders for reconstitution – these are less stable and require the addition of a diluent (normally water for injection or sodium chloride) before using (e.g. Flucloxacillin).

- Powders with the diluent provided – these are fairly unstable and require a specific diluent provided by the manufacturer to reconstitute (e.g. Rifampicin).

- Non-aqueous solutions.

Activity 6.3

Think about the safety features your healthcare provider has introduced to reduce the risk of mistakes in prescribing, preparing or administering IV therapy. (For instance, do you use ready-to-use preparations, needle-free systems, etc.) Identify whether these policies have made any difference to improving practice, and reducing clinical incidents.

Withdrawing solution from an ampoule into a syringe

Ampoules will always pose a risk because of the possibility of contamination from particles (Dougherty 2002). Glass fragments can enter the ampoule when it is broken open, or cause sharps injury to the healthcare practitioner.

Adhere to the following points to ensure safe practice when withdrawing solution from an ampoule into a syringe:

- Use aseptic non-touch technique (ANTT) at all times.

- Tap the ampoule gently to dislodge any medicine contained in the neck of the ampoule.

- Snap open the ampoule using an ampoule snapper.

- Attach a filter needle to the syringe and draw up the required volume of fluid, tilting the ampoule if required. (If the ampoule contains a suspension, it should be gently moved to mix the contents before they are drawn into the syringe.)

See Figures 6.10, 6.11.

- Invert the syringe to remove air bubbles at the needle end. Expel air carefully.

- Exchange the needle. You are now ready to administer the solution using a bolus method. If you are using an intermittent infusion method, the solution will need to be added to diluent fluid.

- Keep the ampoule until the medication has been administered safely.

NB: If you are using a plastic ampoule, some are designed to connect directly to the syringe after the top has been twisted off.

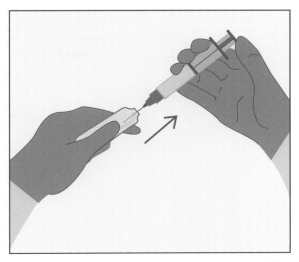

Figure 6.10 Draw up the required volume of fluid

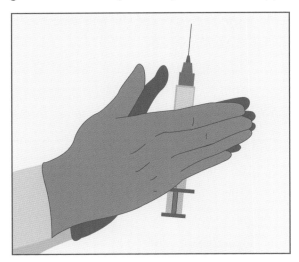

Figure 6.11 Agitate the syringe to mix the contents

Withdrawing a solution or suspension from a vial into a syringe

Vials are associated with potential contamination due to the risk of fragments of the rubber stopper being cut out by the needle (Dougherty 2002). Adhere to the following guidelines to ensure safe practice when withdrawing solution or suspension from a vial into a syringe:

● Use aseptic non-touch technique (ANNT) at all times. Remove the tamper seal from the vial and wipe the rubber stopper with a 2% chlorhexidine gluconate in 70% isopropyl alcohol wipe.

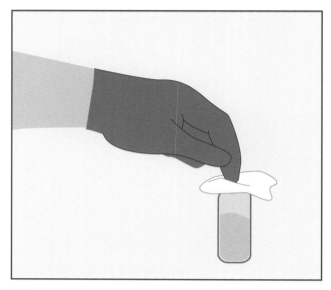

Figure 6.12 Remove the seal from the vial and wipe the rubber stopper

● Allow to dry for a minimum of 30 seconds.

● Attach a filter needle to a syringe. With the needle remaining covered, draw up a volume of air that is equivalent to the required volume of solution to be drawn up.

● Remove the needle cover and insert the needle into the vial through the rubber stopper.

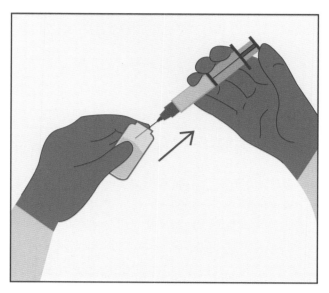

Figure 6.13 Withdraw solution from the vial

- Invert the vial, keeping the filter needle in the solution, and slowly depress the plunger to push air into the vial.
- Release the plunger so that the solution flows into the syringe. (If the vial contains a suspension, it should be gently moved to mix the contents before they are drawn into the syringe.)
- With the vial still attached, invert the syringe. Tap the syringe lightly to remove air bubbles at the filter needle end.
- Fill the syringe with the required volume of solution, and withdraw the filter needle from the syringe.
- Remove the needle, and exchange the needle. You are now ready to administer the solution using a bolus method. If you are using an intermittent infusion method, the solution will need to be added to diluent fluid.

Reconstituting powder from a vial and drawing the resulting suspension or solution into a syringe

Adhere to the following points to ensure safe practice when withdrawing solution or suspension from a vial into a syringe:

- Use ANTT at all times.
- Remove the tamper seal from the vial and wipe the rubber stopper with a 2% chlorhexidine gluconate in 70% isopropyl alcohol wipe.
- Allow to dry for a minimum of 30 seconds.
- Withdraw the required volume of diluent from the syringe.
- Inject the diluent into the vial. Keep the tip of the needle above the solution in the vial, and release the plunger. The syringe will fill with air, which has been displaced by the solution. (If the contents were packed in a vacuum, the solution will be drawn into the vial, and no air will be displaced.)
- With the syringe and needle in place, gently move the vial to mix the contents and dissolve all powder. This may take a few minutes.
- Withdraw the required volume of solution into the syringe.
- Remove the needle, and exchange the needle. You are now ready to administer the solution using a bolus method. If you are using an intermittent infusion method, the solution will need to be added to diluent fluid.

Administering IV medication

Once you have prepared the medication according to the above instructions, you are ready to administer it. The general procedure is explained below; some of the steps will vary slightly depending on the required method of administration.

Table 6.2 Administration of medication using the bolus method

What is done	Why it's done
1. Collect all the equipment required. Medication as prepared, 5mL sodium chloride 0.9% flush (prepared in a 10mL syringe), according to the prescription.	To ensure that the practitioner is prepared, and that the procedure can be carried out quickly and effectively.
2. Wash your hands with soap and water, and apply the principles of ANTT.	To avoid contamination from the healthcare practitioner.
3. Make sure that your second checker is with you to check the prescription, and that you have identified the correct patient.	To ensure that you have the correct patient (NPSA 2006).
4. Obtain consent from the patient, explain the procedure to them and obtain consent	To ensure that the patient is fully informed and agrees to the procedure.
5. Administer flush as required.	To ensure that the line is patent.
6. Administer medication via a needle-free port at the recommended rate (or via a needleless injection cap).	To ensure that the medication is administered at the correct rate.
7. Monitor the patient's clinical condition, either visually or using specific monitoring equipment during the administration.	To ensure that any adverse reaction can be identified, and appropriate and timely actions are taken.
8. Provide patient reassurance throughout the procedure.	To keep the patient calm and relaxed.
9. Complete the procedure, and flush the PVAD.	To reduce the risk of cross contamination and to ensure that the medication is completely administered.
10. Dispose of sharps and other contaminated equipment (as per local healthcare provider's policy).	To reduce the risk of cross contamination.

11. Document the administration on the patient's prescription chart. Complete the patient's notes, recording any problems noted and any actions taken.	To provide a comprehensive record for all healthcare professionals.
12. Ensure that the patient is monitored on an ongoing basis (depending upon the medicine administered and its expected therapeutic effect).	To ensure patient safety and to ensure that any adverse reaction can be identified, and appropriate and timely actions taken.

Adding a prepared medicine to infusion fluid

Once you have prepared the injectable medication, you will need to add it to IV fluid if you intend to administer the medication using either an intermittent or a continuous infusion method.

Points for your practice

Adhere to the following points for practice:

- Use ANTT at all times.
- Prepare the medication in a syringe using one of the methods detailed above.
- Check the outer wrapper of the infusion container. Discard if there are any signs of tampering or damage.
- Where necessary, remove the tamper seal on the additive port according to the manufacturer's instructions, or wipe the rubber stopper with a 2% chlorhexidine gluconate in 70% isopropyl alcohol wipe. Allow to dry for at least 30 seconds.
- Inject the medicine into the infusion container through the centre of the injection port, taking care to avoid puncturing the infusion container or yourself. Withdraw the needle and invert the container to ensure that it is fully mixed prior to starting the infusion.

See Figure 6.14, page 58

- Check the overall appearance of the infusion; ensure that there are no particles, cloudiness or discolouration. Discard if any concerns are noted.
- Label the infusion as per your healthcare provider's guidelines, and administer immediately.

See Figure 6.15, page 58

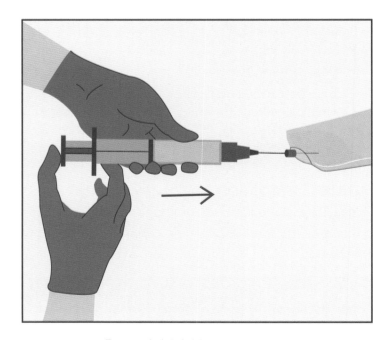

Figure 6.14 Adding a medicine

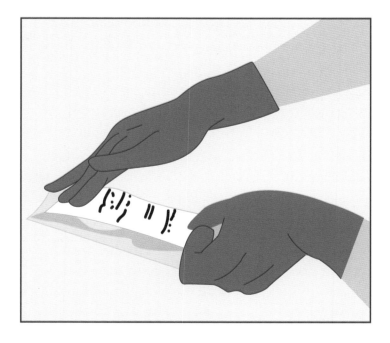

Figure 6.15 Label the infusion

Table 6.3 Administering medicines using an intermittent or continuous infusion method

What is done	Why it's done
1. Collect all the equipment required. Medication as prepared, prescribed fluid, suitable IV administration set, 5mL sodium chloride 0.9% flush, according to the prescription.	To ensure that the practitioner is prepared, and that the procedure can be carried out quickly and effectively.
2. Wash your hands with soap and water, and apply the principles of ANTT.	To avoid contamination from the healthcare practitioner.
3. Make sure that your second checker is with you to check the prescription, and that you have identified the correct patient.	To ensure that you have the correct patient (NPSA 2006).
4. Obtain consent from the patient, explain the procedure to them and obtain consent.	To ensure that the patient is fully informed and agrees to the procedure.
5. Administer flush as required.	To ensure that that the line is patent.
6. Check the administration rate with your second checker. Prepare the infusion and run the fluid through to the end of the infusion line. Connect the additive fluid or the syringe to the needle-free cap using an aseptic technique.	To ensure that appropriate safety checks are completed prior to administration, and that medication is administered at the correct rate.
7. Administer the medicine at the prescribed rate. Use an infusion pump if required.	To ensure that the medication is administered correctly, as per the manufacturer's recommended instructions
8. Monitor the patient's clinical condition, either visually or using specific monitoring equipment during the administration.	To ensure that any adverse reaction can be identified, and appropriate and timely actions can be taken.
9. Document the administration on the patient's prescription chart. Complete the patient's notes, recording any problems noted and any actions taken. Label the infusion line with the date and time of commencement.	To provide a comprehensive record, for other healthcare practitioners.
10. Dispose of sharps and other contaminated equipment (as per local healthcare provider's policy). Wash hands.	To reduce the risk of cross contamination.

11. Once the infusion has completed, flush the PVAD with 5mL sodium chloride 0.9%, and apply a needle-free cap to the access device. Using ANTT, dispose of the infusion line and equipment (as per local healthcare provider's policy).	To ensure patency of the device, and to reduce the risk of infection.

Summary

This chapter has shown that IV therapy is an effective method of delivering both fluids and medication directly into the patient's circulatory system. A step-by-step approach has been provided for the different methods of IV administration. Always ensure that you have read your own healthcare provider's policy and guidelines to familiarise yourself with local practices, and that you are competent to perform the procedure. The risks of intravenous therapy are discussed in Chapter 8, and should be understood alongside the administration techniques.

Chapter 7

Using an infusion device

Learning outcomes

At the end of this chapter, the practitioner will be able to:

- **Select an appropriate infusion device**
- **Reduce risk for the patient during intravenous therapy**
- **Deliver safe intravenous therapy using infusion devices.**

Introduction

There are several different types of infusion pump available, such as volumetric infusion pumps (used to deliver fluid from a bag or other container) and syringe drivers (used to deliver fluid from a syringe). An infusion pump is always recommended to maintain a high degree of accuracy in the administration of intravenous (IV) fluids or medicines.

The healthcare practitioner's responsibilities regarding infusion pumps

The healthcare practitioner responsible for administration needs to ensure that an appropriate infusion pump is used, that it is in good working order, and that they know how to operate it correctly. Your local healthcare provider may insist that you undertake additional training and be competent in the use of the specific devices used within your clinical area. Education and training should ensure that the user understands the basic principles associated with operating infusion pumps, as well as providing practical training in the use of specific devices (Amoore & Adamson 2003).

If you have not been trained, or are not confident in setting up a particular type of infusion pump, *always ask*! All qualified healthcare practitioners are accountable and responsible for their own practice. This means that you are answerable to your professional body and your employer for all your actions and omissions, regardless of the advice or directions given by another professional. Many reported adverse incidents have been due to human error and/ or a lack of understanding of infusion device operation (Amoore & Ingram 2002) so it is essential to adhere to safe practice.

Different types of infusion pump

The main types of infusion are:

- Drip rate controllers
- Volumetric pumps
- Syringe pumps
- Patient controlled analgesia (PCA) pumps.

Drip rate controllers

These are very simple systems that are generally used to administer IV fluid. The infusion rate is selected in drops per minute. The flow is gravity fed, rather than by a forced pump action.

Volumetric pumps

These are the preferred type of infusion pump for administering medium- or large-volume infusions. The infusion rate is selected in millilitres per hour (usually from 1mL to 999mL per hour). For any infusion that needs to be delivered with a rate of less than 5 millilitres per hour, a syringe pump should be used.

Syringe pumps

Syringe pumps are designed to infuse low flow rates. They deliver fluid in millilitres per hour (usually 1mL to 999mL per hour). Syringe pumps will accept different sizes and different brands of syringe; some of the newer models automatically detect the syringe size and type. Syringe pumps should not be used for rates less than 0.5mL per hour for adult patients, as an increase in the occlusion response time occurs.

Patient controlled analgesia (PCA) pumps

Patient controlled analgesia (PCA) pumps are similar to syringe pumps. However, the pump has the facility to enable patients to self-administer a bolus dose of the medication themselves. The PCA pump has different programming options, which need to be set by the relevant healthcare professional.

Choosing the right infusion pump

Before a decision is made on which pump to use, consider:

● Is the patient a neonate, child or adult?

● What sort of infusion is required?

● Does the patient have special needs?

● Is there a critical volume that needs to be delivered?

● If the infusion stopped for any reason, would this be dangerous?

Using infusion pumps

When safely used, infusion devices can deliver fluid or medication in a controlled manner, and are relatively straightforward to use. The basic operation of an infusion pump involves setting up the pump to deliver the fluid at the prescribed rate over a specified period of time.

All infusion pumps feature the following characteristics:

● A method to generate pressure to infuse fluid

● A method of controlling the infusion rate

● A fluid container (syringe or bag)

● Tubing that allows the fluid container to be attached to the patient. Infusion lines will generally be manufactured specifically for a certain pump and you must always ensure that the set designed for that particular pump is used. (NB: Standard infusion giving sets should not be used.)

Activity 7.1

Look at the different types of infusion pumps that are available to use in your own clinical area. Familiarise yourself with how each type of pump works, and the functions and features that are on that particular device.

To work effectively, infusion pumps must generate a higher amount of pressure to overcome the lower level of pressure which is present along both the administration set and the patient's own venous pressure. The pressure in an adult vein is between 25 and 80mmHg (Boyd 2013). For the fluid/medication to flow into the vein, the pressure must be higher than this.

Once the higher pressure is generated, this enables the fluid or medication to be delivered into the patient's circulatory system. Syringe pumps generate a higher pressure through a motor, which applies force to drive the syringe plunger forward. In volumetric pumps, pressure is generated through the squeezing of administration sets.

Points for your practice

Q. How is a higher amount of pressure achieved in an infusion using a gravity fed infusion system?

A. A higher amount of pressure will be achieved when the fluid bag is higher than the infusion site. The pressure will be higher due to gravity, and will 'push' fluid into the vein.

All infusion pumps have the ability to generate a high level of pressure; pressure-limiting methods are therefore needed (Amoore & Adamson 2003). These compare pressure in the administration set to a pre-set limit, known as an occlusion alarm pressure. If the pressure limit is exceeded, then the fluid delivery will stop, and the infusion pump will activate an alarm (Amoore & Adamson 2003). The alarm limit may be fixed, or variable according to the infusion rate, or sometimes it can be adjusted by the user. Problems with infusion pump alarms will be discussed later in this chapter (see p. 67).

An accurate level of fluid delivery is essential to ensure safe practice when using infusion pumps. Infusion pumps can control the pumping mechanism to control the infusion rate; however, they do not measure the rate. Volumetric pumps work by accurately squeezing a precise part of the infusion set at a determined frequency necessary to deliver the required infusion rate. A syringe pump works by controlling the infusion rate by driving forward the plunger at the required rate.

Human error is a common cause of inaccurate infusion rates, for one or more of the following reasons:

- Prescription error
- Incorrect setting by user

- Failure to set the flow rate
- Lack of understanding of the device operation
- Device tampering or device faults.

When setting up the pump, always remember to purge the line before commencing the infusion. Purging the line involves running the fluid or medication through the line before it is connected to the patient. Many of the latest infusion pumps will do this automatically for you, by simply pressing a button. This will allow the purging to be performed when the giving set or syringe is mounted in the pump.

When using syringe drivers, the purge function will remove any backlash, meaning that the IV therapy will be delivered to the patient as soon as the infusion starts. Backlash only occurs with syringe drivers, and it happens because it may take some time for the pump to take up the slack in the system. This can cause a delay in administration to the patient (particularly if the infusion rate is slow).

A useful feature of infusion pumps is the ability to administer an extra volume of medication (known as a bolus dose) in addition to the continuous infusion. This is a standard feature of many infusion pumps, and is commonly seen with patient controlled analgesia (PCA) pumps. For other infusion device systems, the bolus method is often only used within critical care environments.

Many infusion pumps deliver fluid in millilitres per hour, and will automatically work out the infusion flow rate for you. The formula that is used to check the infusion rate calculation is:

$$\text{Infusion rate} = \frac{\text{amount of fluid (mL)}}{\text{Infusion time (hours)}}$$

Chapter 4 provides detailed information on the calculation of infusion rates, as well as general medication calculations, so look through that chapter if you need to refresh your knowledge.

When an infusion ends, the infusion pump will run at a very slow rate (normally around 2mL per hour). This is known as the 'keep vein open' (KVO) rate. It is used to prevent the venous access from becoming blocked, and prevents blood from clotting.

Potential complications when using infusion pumps

Infusion pumps have some general features to improve their safety, and to make them easier for users to operate. For instance, most volumetric pumps have alarms that will sound to notify the user that there is a problem with the infusion pump. There are also anti-tamper features (such as button locks) to prevent unauthorised changing of the controls or device tampering. Patient controlled analgesia (PCA) pumps also have a physical lock and key to prevent unauthorised access to the infusion pump controls and the fluid container.

Activity 7.2

List the checks that you make when setting up an infusion. Why do you undertake these checks? Explain your reason for each one.

Infusion-related problems

There are many infusion-related problems, the most common of which are detailed below. You will need to ensure that you are aware of what to do in the event of a problem with the infusion pump.

Air in line

The presence of air in the infusion line is a significant concern. This is potentially dangerous for the patient, and must be avoided. When a pump is set up correctly, it is easy to minimise the 'air in line' alarm. Although manufacturers do their best to minimise the amount of air in infusion bags, there will always be some present, as air dissolves in fluid, and the pumping action of the infusion pump itself will release air. Most infusion pumps will detect air in the giving set (with the exception of syringe infusion pumps), and will accordingly sound an alarm to alert the user.

Uncontrolled free flow

Free flow is the uncontrolled flow of fluid from an intravenous bag or syringe. Free flow can occur with all types of infusion pump, and it is potentially dangerous because it can cause overdose of medication or over-infusion of fluid. The most common example of free flow occurring is when a practitioner has left the roller clamp open on the infusion line, or they have forgotten to close the clamp when removing the infusion set from a pump. When opening the door of an infusion device, the roller clamp *must* be closed – or the device will free flow.

It is also possible to get free flow from a syringe infusion device – in two ways. Firstly, if the syringe is higher than the giving set, the pressure in the syringe will be higher than at the end of the infusion line. This pressure may be sufficient to push forward the plunger on the syringe. Secondly, free flow can happen if the syringe being used is damaged. Air can enter around the seal between the plunger and the syringe barrel. If the syringe is higher than the infusion site this can cause the plunger to move, causing free flow.

It is important to note that both these risks can be minimised by reducing the height between the syringe and the infusion site.

Points for your practice

Always ensure that the clamp on a syringe is clamped off to prevent free flow. Also, be careful when disconnecting or removing a syringe. At this point, it is easy to raise the syringe in the air, which could potentially cause free flow.

Occlusion alarms

How soon an alarm sounds depends on the speed of the infusion, as well as the pressure setting on the infusion pump. All alarms indicate a problem with the infusion pump, and should be acted upon in the first instance.

Common triggers for infusion alarms include:

- A blockage in the line (which can be caused by leaving the roller clamp closed)
- A blocked PVAD
- A patient bending an arm
- The use of a small-gauge cannula, which has a high flow rate
- The alarm limit being set too low.

There are hazards caused by an occlusion, such as an interruption of the intended therapy. The patient may also inadvertently receive a bolus dose of medication or fluid once the occlusion is removed. This can potentially cause over-administration of the prescribed medication, which can be hazardous for the patient. Many of the latest infusion device models have a sophisticated 'back off' mechanism. When an occlusion is detected, they reverse the administration and suck some of the bolus back into the syringe, thus minimising the amount received by the patient.

Summary

This chapter has identified the different types of infusion pumps that can be used in various healthcare settings. You will now understand how to choose the most appropriate pump to use. You will also recognise the standard features of infusion pumps, be able to identify potential problems with their use, and know how to guard against such problems occurring.

Chapter 8

Risk, complications and adverse reactions

Learning outcomes

At the end of this chapter, the practitioner will be able to:

- **Identify the key risks and complications related to intravenous therapy**
- **Recognise the implications for clinical practice.**

Introduction

There are numerous risks and complications identified with intravenous (IV) therapy. The key risks and complications are identified below so that you are aware of what to do in the event of a problem.

Anaphylaxis

Anaphylaxis is an immediate systemic hypersensitivity reaction caused by an immunological release of mediators from mast cells and basophils (Ingram & Lavery 2005). It can have life-threatening consequences for an individual. The causative factors of anaphylaxis include medicines, foods, insect stings, and latex and radio-contrast media. Anaphylaxis is often predictable, so it is important to identify how to decrease risks (Ingram & Lavery 2005), and consider factors such as:

- Patient history
- The route of IV therapy administration, and the rate at which medication/fluid is administered

- Any known allergies or previous history of anaphylaxis
- Any medication contraindications, if there is a known history of anaphylaxis. This requires a good level of medication knowledge.

Reactions due to anaphylaxis range from a mild skin reaction to cardiovascular collapse. The actions required depend on the severity of the symptoms present.

Points for your practice

If anaphylaxis is suspected, take the following actions:

- Discontinue the medicine immediately
- Summon emergency help and assistance
- Administer oxygen, IV fluids and adrenaline
- Check airway, breathing, circulation (ABC)
- Start cardiopulmonary resuscitation (CPR) if there is no pulse present
- Monitor vital signs, ECG and oxygen saturations.

If the patient is conscious, the healthcare practitioner will need to provide reassurance, communicate effectively and provide information and education. Drain and Volcheck (2001) recommend that observation is required for a minimum of 2 hours, and in severe cases up to 24 hours.

Speed shock

Speed shock is a systemic reaction that occurs when a substance foreign to the body is introduced rapidly (Weinstein & Hagle 2014). It is a particular hazard when administering medication using a peripheral venous access device (PVAD) or a bolus method of administration. To avoid speed shock, the practitioner must ensure that the IV fluid or medication is administered at the prescribed rate. When flushing a PVAD, a 'push pause' method should be used (an alternating stop start technique) (Ingram & Lavery 2005). The use of an infusion device is also recommended – to regulate the fluid flow into the circulatory system.

Circulatory overload

Circulatory overload occurs when a volume of IV fluid is given too rapidly. Venous pressure increases and creates the potential for cardiac dilution and pulmonary oedema (Dougherty

2002). Circulatory overload can result in congestive cardiac failure, shock and cardiac arrest. Particular groups at risk include the elderly, those with already impaired cardiac or renal function and children. To avoid circulatory overload, the use of infusion devices is recommended to ensure that the infusion is delivered at the prescribed rate. A sound knowledge of the medication and the rate of administration is also crucial to ensure safe practice.

Free flow

Free flow is the uncontrolled flow of fluid from an IV bag or syringe. Free flow can occur with all types of infusions, and it is potentially dangerous because it can cause overdose of medication or over-infusion of fluid. The most common example of free flow occurring is when a practitioner has left the roller clamp open on the infusion line, or they have forgotten to close the clamp when removing the infusion set from a pump. When opening the door of an infusion device, the roller clamp *must* be closed – or the device will free flow.

It is also possible to get free flow from a syringe infusion device – in two ways (see Chapter 7, p. 66).

Infection

Staphylococcus epidermidis is a type of skin-based bacteria that can enter the circulatory system through the access device insertion site. Other bacteria (such as *Staphylococcus aureus, Candida* species and *Enterococci*) can be introduced through contaminated infusion fluid (McCallum 2012), causing systemic bacteraemia. Once micro-organisms are introduced into contaminated infusion fluid, they collect and grow on both living and inert substances. This is known as a biofilm. If the biofilm fragments dislodge and enter the patient's circulatory system, this can cause bacteraemia or sepsis, which can have potentially devastating consequences for the patient. Sepsis can compromise the patient's quality of life, or even be fatal, as well as increasing healthcare costs, due to a more prolonged hospital stay.

Fungaemia is the presence of fungi or yeasts in the blood. The most common type is caused by Candida species. It is most commonly seen in immunosuppressed patients with severe neutropenia, cancer patients, or patients with IV devices. Symptoms can range from mild to extreme and are similar to flu-like symptoms. Other symptoms may include pain, acute confusion, infections and chronic fatigue. Skin infections can include persistent or non-healing wounds and lesions, sweating, itching and unusual discharge or drainage. It is often difficult to diagnose fungaemia because routine blood cultures often have a poor sensitivity.

Infections resulting from IV therapy can cover a wide range of symptoms from a minor irritation at the site (local infection) to increased morbidity and mortality (Ingram & Lavery

2005). Infections can be divided into two main groups – exogenous and endogenous. Exogenous infections occur when micro-organisms exist and originate outside the patient's body. A typical example of an exogenous infection is one that is created due to cross-contamination from the healthcare practitioner or equipment used (Ingram & Lavery 2005). Both types of infections can occur through intrinsic or extrinsic contamination. Intrinsic sources of infection are present in equipment or the medication prior to use (e.g. when packaging has been damaged). Extrinsic infection is introduced during use (e.g. bottle or bag changes, when adding to infusion fluid).

Points for your practice

What are the signs and symptoms of local and systemic infection?

Signs and symptoms are erythema (reddening of the skin), swelling, pus, warmth to the area and pain, ranging to fever, malaise, tachycardia, hypotension, shock and death if the infection spreads systemically. Infection prevention needs to be an integral part of the healthcare practitioner's role, and it is essential that good handwashing practice and a strict aseptic technique is adhered to when dealing with an IV device, as this significantly reduces the risk of extrinsic infection.

Phlebitis

Phlebitis is defined as inflammation of the vein (specifically the Tunica Intima part of the vein), and is characterised by redness, pain and swelling (Dougherty 2008). It is estimated that up to 80% of patients receiving IV therapy have reported signs and symptoms of phlebitis (Ung, Cook, *et al.* 2002), showing that it is a common problem within clinical practice. There are three types of phlebitis – mechanical, infective and chemical. Phlebitis can be prevented by careful selection of the vein and the device, and use of an aseptic non-touch technique (ANTT) when inserting and caring for IV access devices.

Mechanical phlebitis happens when the device itself causes inflammation in the Tunica Intima section of the vein. To reduce the risk of mechanical phlebitis, it is recommended that the smallest-gauge PVAD is inserted (Scales 2005). Changing the device every 72 hours also reduces the risk (RCN 2010).

Infective phlebitis is caused by micro-organisms entering the vein through the insertion site. It can be attributed to poor intravenous cannulation technique, or it can be a consequence of the practitioner's poor hand hygiene practices. Micro-organisms can also originate from the patient's own skin flora, or via cross contamination through injectable ports on the IV access device. It is important that healthcare practitioners adopt ANTT when inserting a PVAD, and also part of good intravenous access device care to reduce the risk of infection.

Chemical phlebitis is caused by the administered fluid or medication causing inflammation in the vein. This can be due to the irritant nature of the medication being administered – the pH and osmolality (concentration) of the medication. For example, strong alkaline, acidic or hypertonic drugs can cause irritation if injected into a small vein with an insufficient blood flow (Ingram & Lavery 2005). If you are administering fluid or medication, it is vital that the correct strength of infusion is prepared before administration begins. Medication for IV administration should be prepared and administered according to the manufacturer's guidelines, and according to your local healthcare provider's policy and procedure.

The common signs and symptoms of phlebitis often include erythema (a reddening of the skin) and swelling along the vein. This then leads to an eventual hardening of the vein and a 'cord-like' appearance. The area will feel warm, and the patient may feel pain or discomfort during administration of fluid or medicines (Higginson 2011).

Many local healthcare providers use a phlebitis scale to assist practitioners as part of daily IV access device care and as a checking and recording procedure. Although various phlebitis scales have been published, the Royal College of Nursing (2010) have adopted Jackson (1998) as the preferred risk assessment tool. This includes a scoring system ranging from 0 (no signs of phlebitis) to 5 (advanced stage thrombophlebitis); and provides the practitioner with a management plan, depending upon the patient's score. The management plan includes removal of the device, as well as symptom control – if early indications of phlebitis are present.

In an attempt to reduce the incidence of IV device associated infections, and to improve compliance with effective record keeping and documentation, the Department of Health (2011) advocates the use of a visual phlebitis tool as a care bundle for PVAD care.

Table 8.1 Phlebitis scoring system (adapted from Jackson 1998)

Clinical signs	Phlebitis score	What to do
IV access device site appears healthy	0	Observe site
One of the following is reported: • Pain at IV access device site • Redness around IV access device site	1	Observe site (clinical signs may signify early indicators of phlebitis)

Clinical signs	Phlebitis score	What to do
Two of the following are reported: • Pain at IV access device site • Erythema (reddening of the skin) around the IV access device site • Swelling around the IV access device site	2	Re-site IV access device (clinical signs signify first signs of phlebitis)
All the following are reported, and evident: • Pain along the path of the access device • Erythema • Induration	3	Re-site IV access device and consider treatment (clinical signs signify medium stage of phlebitis)
All the following are reported, and evident: • Pain along the path of the access device • Erythema • Induration • Palpable venous cord (feels like a hardened cord along the vein)	4	Re-site IV access device and consider treatment (may signify advanced thrombophlebitis or early signs of thrombophlebitis)
All the following are reported, and evident: • Pain along the path of the access device • Erythema • Induration • Palpable venous cord (feels like a hardened cord along the vein) • Pyrexia	5	Re-site IV access device and implement treatment (clinical signs signify advanced stage of thrombophlebitis)

Early phlebitis at a PVAD site usually resolves after the device is removed or re-sited (Higginson 2011). The initial treatment aim is to stop any infusion running, and to remove or re-site the IV access device if the patient has a score of 2 or above (Jackson 1998). However, it is important to consider the patient's needs at this point. For example, a new PVAD should be sited as soon as possible, to avoid any delay in treatment. The affected limb should be elevated to minimise inflammation (Reis 2009) and anti-inflammatory analgesia can be prescribed and administered to treat the inflammation and pain associated with phlebitis (Higginson 2011).

Infiltration and extravasation

Infiltration and extravasation is more commonly known as intravenous PVAD 'tissuing'. Although this is not an officially accepted term, you may still hear it used in the clinical practice setting. Infiltration is the inadvertent administration of a non-vesicant fluid or medication into surrounding tissues; whereas extravasation is the inadvertent administration of a vesicant (chemical) fluid or solution into the surrounding tissues. Examples of vesicant medications include Vancomycin, potassium chloride and dopamine.

Signs and symptoms of infiltration and extravasation include swelling at the insertion site, cooling and blanching of the skin, and leakage around the device. The patient may complain of pain, usually related to the amount of swelling at the insertion site. Extravasation can appear as redness around the affected site, similar to sunburn.

If the patient complains of a burning-type sensation, they will need to be assessed and treated immediately, as tissue necrosis could occur. Tissue necrosis can lead to long-term problems, sometimes resulting in the necrotic tissue having to be surgically removed. The degree of tissue damage will depend on the type of drug or fluid being infused and how long it is present in the tissues before being discovered. Both infiltration and extravasation usually cause the slowing or stopping of the infusion, which is often the first sign that there is a problem with a PVAD.

Treatment options for infiltration and extravasation should be commenced at the first sign of a problem. If an IV medication or fluid is running, it should be stopped immediately. If IV therapy is to be maintained, the PVAD should be re-sited on another upper limb.

Infiltration and extravasation are often caused by poor IV site selection, especially if the device is inserted over a point of flexion. A traumatic insertion can cause damage to the Tunica Intima (lining) of the vein, thus predisposing it to further damage when an irritating fluid or medication is infused. In addition, inadequate securing of the device predisposes it to move, which can potentially cause the tip to go through the vein wall, thus infusing medication or fluid into the surrounding tissues.

Sharps injuries

'Sharps' are needles, blades (such as scalpels) and other medical instruments that could cause an injury by cutting or pricking the skin. A sharps injury is an incident in which a needle, blade (such as scalpel) or other medical instrument penetrates the skin. This is sometimes called a percutaneous injury. These types of injuries are a well-known risk in the health and social care sector.

Sharps contaminated with an infected patient's blood can transmit more than 20 diseases, including Hepatitis B, C and Human Immunodeficiency Virus (HIV). Because of this transmission risk, sharps injuries can cause worry and stress to the many thousands of practitioners who receive them. It is vital that all healthcare staff performing clinical procedures adhere to their local healthcare provider's policies, and professionally update themselves by reading recent evidence-based guidelines, and reflecting upon their current practice.

The EU directive for Safer Sharps (Health and Safety Executive 2013) has made several recommendations in order to prevent sharps injuries from occurring:

- Sharps handling should be kept to a minimum.
- Needles must not be bent or broken prior to disposal.
- Needles and sharps must not be disassembled prior to disposal.
- Needles should not be re-capped.
- Used sharps must be discarded into a sharps container at the point of use. Sharps bins must not be filled above two-thirds full (there is a mark on the side of the sharps container indicating the fill line). Containers should not be kept on the floor and should be located in a safe position.
- Consider the use of needle-stick prevention devices to provide greater safety for practitioners. These need to be evaluated in terms of their effectiveness, and the impact of care and cost benefits.

The *Health and Safety (Sharp Instruments in Healthcare) Regulations 2013* can be accessed through www.hse.gov.uk and is a good source of additional reading.

What to do in the event of a sharps-related injury

All local healthcare providers will have their own procedure to follow in the event of a sharps-related incident (frequently known as a needle-stick injury). It is important that you are aware of what to do if you have received this type of injury.

Always look at your local healthcare provider's guidelines to provide you with specific advice for your own area, but the following points will always apply:

- Encourage the wound to bleed and wash it under running water.
- Report the incident to the manager or person in charge.
- Report to your Occupational Health department within 24 hours where possible (allow longer for weekends and bank holidays). They will tell you whether blood needs taking from your patient and you, if there is a risk of infection to you. Consent will be needed to take bloods from your patient.
- If you are concerned and your Occupational Health department is not open, go to A&E (especially if your patient is thought to have hepatitis or HIV).
- Once immediate first-aid measures have been put in place, ensure that you complete a clinical incident form so that the incident can be recorded. You may be asked to write a statement detailing how the needle-stick injury occurred. Make sure you document the incident while it is fresh in your memory.

Reporting incidents

A medication incident is described as an event or omission arising during clinical care that has caused physical or psychological injury to a patient (Dougherty 2002). A near miss is described as a situation or event that has failed to develop due to a result of action, thus preventing harm (DH 2000). Common causes of incidents (and near misses) can include workplace stress, limited or insufficient staff education, or miscommunication – through illegible prescriptions, medicines with similar names or overuse of abbreviations (DH 2000). Incidents do unfortunately sometimes occur, and – although fairly rare – they can have serious implications and may be very distressing for both healthcare practitioners and patients.

To avoid an incident, it is well worth remembering the '5 Rs' checklist (Clayton 1987, see also p. 32) as well as ensuring that the person preparing and administering the medication is completely satisfied. Do not simply rely on a second checker to confirm your answer. You must always be sure that you can calculate and prepare the medication without relying on the skills of others.

You will need to familiarise yourself with the process for completing an incident form, and the process for reporting – should an untoward incident or near miss occur (particularly out of hours or at the weekend, as procedures may vary). Each healthcare provider will be able to provide you with specific information on this to ensure that incident reporting is completed effectively. You will need to provide full details, including date, time and place of the incident, the people involved (staff and/or patients), a description of how the incident occurred, and what actions were taken. This may include the submission of a statement providing additional information.

The incident may be investigated; this is an important part of the process so that lessons can be learnt to ensure that similar mistakes are not made again. Some healthcare practitioners are nervous about reporting incidents, due to fear of blame or disciplinary action. However, it is important that all healthcare providers provide an open atmosphere and are supportive of staff (DH 2000). Reflection should be encouraged so that untoward events are reported and any systemic errors can be identified and resolved (Dougherty 2002).

Summary

This chapter has identified some of the risks that need to be considered when preparing and administering IV therapy. Always make sure that you adhere to your local health provider's infection prevention and control procedures to ensure your safety as well as your patients'. You will also need to familiarise yourself with the correct procedures to follow if an incident occurs.

Chapter 9

Professional responsibilities

Learning outcomes

At the end of this chapter, the practitioner will be able to:

- **Understand the training and development required to administer intravenous therapy safely and effectively**
- **Understand the professional requirements associated with the administration of intravenous therapy.**

Most healthcare providers have a specific system for training their staff in intravenous therapy (Whyte 2001). This may be in the form of attendance at a study day, an e-learning package or a competency-based workbook. The healthcare practitioner will need to demonstrate an appropriate level of knowledge and have an assessed level of competence prior to undertaking this role. Appendices 1, 2 and 3 at the back of this book give guidance on recording your competence schedule in administering IV medication. In addition to any local training that is offered, healthcare practitioners also need to be aware of and maintain specific legal and professional requirements to undertake the role.

Most healthcare providers require healthcare practitioners to attend a formal study day, comprising (O'Hanlon *et al.* 2008):

- Anatomy and physiology
- Consideration of the legal and professional issues

- Professional responsibility and accountability through the professional code of practice
- Pharmacology and calculating medication doses
- Care and maintenance of central venous catheters (CVCs) and peripheral venous access devices (PVADs)
- Preparation and administration of intravenous (IV) medication
- Practical demonstration of the procedure
- The key risks and complications associated with IV therapy.

Some healthcare providers require attendance on an annual IV therapy update, where practitioners are formally assessed on their knowledge, receive updates on good practice and an open forum is provided to address any queries.

In terms of professional requirements, practitioners will always need to familiarise themselves with any local guidelines and procedures that are in place, and ensure that they are followed at all times. As a practitioner, you must always remember the principles of safe administration of medicines. As stated by the Nursing and Midwifery Council (2008), the administration of IV medication 'is not solely a mechanical task to be performed on strict compliance with the written prescription … it requires thought and exercise of professional judgement …' (NMC 2008 p. 4).

Healthcare professionals must ensure that they exercise accountability at all stages of medication administration. Accountability for registered healthcare practitioners is integral to the concept of professionalism. Professional regulation through a statutory body (such as the Nursing and Midwifery Council) is required in order to practice professionally. A registered practitioner has professional and legal accountability in four spheres:

- Their professional regulatory body (with the possible penalty of being removed from the register if found to be in breach of their professional code of conduct)
- The patient through civil law (with the possible penalty of being sued through the legal system)
- The employer through the contract of employment
- The public through criminal law (with the possible penalty being criminal prosecution).

Any individual who has been harmed as a result of poor or inadequate care whilst being treated by a registered professional can claim compensation under civil law. The claim may be considered as a breach of the individual practitioner's duty of care.

Activity 9.1

Look up the terms: accountability, duty of care and civil law. What do they mean? How do you think your understanding of these concepts affects your daily practice?

As a healthcare practitioner, in terms of accountability relating to the safe administration of IV therapy, you must:

- Be competent to perform the skill
- Have undergone the correct training
- Have undergone a period of supervised practice
- Have been deemed competent by another competent practitioner in order to perform the skill unsupervised
- Be happy to perform the skill
- Be willing to recognise your own limitations
- Be willing to retrain if you have not performed the skill for an extended period of time
- Be aware of the legal and ethical issues and update your practice accordingly.

Consent

It is vital for the patient to consent to their treatment (assuming they have normal mental capacity). From a legal and professional perspective, it is essential that consent is:

- Given by a competent person
- Given voluntarily
- Informed (i.e. the patient has been given full information about the procedure and any associated risks).

Consent can be given verbally, or it can be implied (e.g. a patient holds out their arm) or it can be written. Currently, there is no legal requirement for consent to be given in a particular way; they are all valid methods. Implied consent should be avoided, as it has no standing in a court of law. It is important that the procedure is fully explained. The potential risks must be identified so that the patient can exercise their right to say no. Whichever method of consent is used, it is essential that it is documented in the patient's notes. If the decision is not to administer medication, this will also need to be recorded on the patient's prescription chart.

Effective record keeping

Effective record keeping is essential in terms of your own accountability as a registered healthcare practitioner (NMC 2015), and to maintain a good standard of professional practice. Failure to document your interventions accurately could have consequences, from both a legal and a professional perspective. Any documentation required for legal or complaints purposes will be carefully scrutinised; and any failure noted could potentially compromise the individual concerned. The importance of documentation is often overlooked within the healthcare profession, particularly when the workload is high. However, when it comes to completing patient records, it is worth remembering the saying 'care not documented is care not done'.

Summary

This chapter has identified some of the fundamental professional responsibilities in relation to your practice. Ensure that you are able to maintain your accountability at all times. Further information on accountability and responsibility can be sourced through your professional body. Speak to your workplace training and development department to ensure that you are familiar with the specific training requirements for your workplace to enable you to practice IV therapy.

Appendix 1

Competency checklist for the preparation of intravenous therapy using a bolus method

Tick under 'Yes' or 'No' for each item on the list, as appropriate.

Key objective	Yes	No
Assessment of the patient:		
• You have accurately assessed the patient, and the need for intravenous therapy has been confirmed.		
• You have gained informed consent from the patient.		
• The IV access device to be used has been inspected (and is patent).		
Preparation:		
• Wash hands thoroughly		
• You have consulted the patient's prescription and have ascertained the following:		
a) Medication		
b) Dose		
c) Date and time of administration		
d) Route and method of administration		
e) Validity of prescription		
f) Prescriber's signature is present.		
• All details are checked with a second checker, as required by your healthcare provider's policy.		

	Yes	No
• The environment is prepared appropriately prior to undertaking the procedure.		
• You have selected the appropriate equipment.		
• The packaging is intact and not damaged.		
• The medication to be administered has been prepared.		
• A Sodium Chloride 0.9% flush has been prepared.		
• All equipment and medication to be administered has been placed in a clinically clean receptacle.		
The procedure:		
• Wash your hands thoroughly.		
• Check and confirm the patient identity against the name band (where appropriate), the prescription, prepared drug. Confirm with second checker (where required).		
• Wash hands thoroughly and put on personal protective equipment (PPE).		
• Stop the infusion (if an infusion is in progress).		
• Place a sterile towel under the insertion site to create a sterile field.		
• Clean the injection port with a 2% chlorhexidine and 70% isopropyl alcohol swab and allow to dry.		
• Inject the flush to ensure PVAD patency.		
• Change syringes and inject the medication smoothly over the required time period.		
• Observe the access site at all times, in case of complications.		
• If more than one medication is to be administered; flush with sodium chloride 0.9%, and repeat the above steps.		

	Yes	No
• At the end of the bolus injection, flush with Sodium Chloride 0.9% and clean the injection port with a 2% chlorhexidine and 70% isopropyl alcohol swab and allow to dry.		
Aftercare:		
• Allow time for the patient to ask questions, and tell them who to report to in case of any noted problems.		
• Ensure that you have left your patient comfortable and relaxed.		
• Record medication administration on the patient's prescription chart (and on the fluid balance chart, where appropriate).		
• Ensure that all clinical waste has been disposed of as per your local healthcare provider's policy.		
• Make sure all sharps have been disposed of as per your local healthcare provider's policy.		
• Remove PPE and wash your hands thoroughly.		

Signature of learner ————————————————————————

(Print name) ————————————————————————————

Signature of assessor ——————————————————————

(Print name) ————————————————————————————

Date of competency ——————————————————————

Appendix 2

Competency checklist for the preparation of intravenous therapy using an intermittent or continuous infusion method

Tick under 'Yes' or 'No' for each item on the list, as appropriate.

Key objective	Yes	No
Assessment of the patient:		
• You have accurately assessed the patient, and the need for intravenous therapy has been confirmed.		
• You have gained informed consent from the patient.		
• The IV access device to be used has been inspected (and is patent).		
Preparation:		
• Wash your hands thoroughly.		
• You have consulted the patient's prescription and have ascertained the following:		
• Medication		
• Dose		
• Date and time of administration		
• Route and method of administration		
• Validity of prescription		
• Prescriber's signature is present.		
• All details are checked with a second checker, as required by your healthcare provider's policy.		

	Yes	No
• The environment is prepared appropriately prior to undertaking the procedure.		
• You have selected the appropriate equipment.		
• The packaging is intact and not damaged.		
• The medication to be administered has been prepared.		
• A Sodium Chloride 0.9% flush has been prepared.		
• All equipment and medication to be administered has been placed in a clinically clean receptacle.		
The procedure:		
• Wash your hands thoroughly.		
• Check and confirm the patient's identity against the name band (where appropriate), as well as the prescription and prepared drug. Confirm with second checker (where required).		
• Prime the intravenous administration set with the infusion fluid and hang it on the infusion stand.		
• Wash your hands thoroughly and put on personal protective equipment (PPE).		
• Place a sterile towel underneath the insertion site to create a sterile field.		
• Clean the injection port with a 2% chlorhexidine and 70% isopropyl alcohol swab and allow to dry.		
• Inject the flush to ensure PVAD patency.		
• Connect the infusion administration set to the patient.		
• Adjust flow rate according to your medication calculations.		

	Yes	No
• Ensure that the administration set is taped into position to ensure that there no strain is placed on the intravenous access device.		
• Observe the access site at all times, in case of complications.		
• Return to the infusion at frequent intervals to ensure constant monitoring.		
Aftercare:		
• Allow time for the patient to ask questions, and tell them who to report to in case of any noted problems.		
• Ensure that you have left your patient comfortable and relaxed.		
• Record medication administration on the patient's prescription chart (and on the fluid balance chart, where appropriate).		
• Ensure that all clinical waste has been disposed of as per your local healthcare provider's policy.		
• Make sure all sharps have been disposed of as per your local healthcare provider's policy.		
• Remove PPE and wash your hands thoroughly.		
Following completion of the infusion:		
• Stop the infusion once all fluid has been delivered.		
• Wash your hands thoroughly and put on PPE.		
• Disconnect the infusion set.		
• Clean the injection port with a 2% chlorhexidine and 70% isopropyl alcohol swab and allow to dry.		
• Ensure that the patient is left comfortable, and is aware of who to contact if any problems are noted.		

	Yes	No
• Ensure all clinical waste has been disposed of as per your local healthcare provider's policy.		
• Make sure all sharps have been disposed of, as per your local healthcare provider's policy.		
• Record the medication administration completion time on the patient's prescription chart (and on the fluid balance chart, where appropriate).		

Signature of learner —————————————————————————

(Print name) ————————————————————————————

Signature of assessor ————————————————————————

(Print name) ————————————————————————————

Date of competency ———————————————————————

Appendix 3

Record of supervised practice

Administration using a bolus method

Practice number/ date	Medication prepared/ administered	Problems/actions taken	Supervisor's signature	Practitioner's signature
Example	*Flucloxacillin 500mg*	*Patient reported pain on administration – VIP score 0 – to monitor access site*	*A. Supervisor*	*A. Practitioner*
1.				
2.				
3.				
4.				
5.				

Administration using an intermittent infusion method

Practice number/ date	Medication prepared/ administered	Problems/actions taken	Supervisor's signature	Practitioner's signature
Example	*Flucloxacillin 500mg*	*Patient reported pain on administration – VIP score 0 – to monitor access site*	*A. Supervisor*	*A. Practitioner*
1.				
2.				
3.				
4.				
5.				

Administration using a continuous infusion method

Practice number/ date	Medication prepared/ administered	Problems/actions taken	Supervisor's signature	Practitioner's signature
Example	Sodium chloride 0.9% (1000mL)		A. Supervisor	A. Practitioner
1.				
2.				
3.				
4.				
5.				

Appendix 4:

Answers to medications calculations from Chapter 4 and Chapter 6

Activity 4.2 Working out the drops per minute

1. 500mL of 5% dextrose is prescribed to be administered over 4 hours. The administration set delivers 20 drops per mL.

- Volume in mL = 500 (as you have a 500mL bag of fluid)
- Time in hours = 4 (as it is to be administered over 4 hours)
- Drops per mL = 20 (as your infusion set delivers 20 drops per mL)

This would work out at:

$$\text{Drops rate per minute} = \frac{500}{4} \times \frac{20}{60}$$

Answer: 41.6 drops per minute (round up to 42)

2. 500mL of whole blood is prescribed to be administered over 4 hours. The administration set delivers 15 drops per mL.

- Volume in mL = 500 (as you have a 500mL bag of fluid)
- Time in hours = 4 (as it is to be administered over 4 hours)
- Drops per mL = 15 (as your infusion set delivers 15 drops per mL)

This would work out at:

$$\text{Drops rate per minute} = \frac{500}{4} \times \frac{15}{60}$$

Answer: 31.25 drops per minute (round down to 31)

3. 1000mL of Hartmann's solution is prescribed to be administered over 6 hours. The administration set delivers 20 drops per mL.

- Volume in mL = 1000 (as you have a 1000mL bag of fluid)
- Time in hours = 6 (as it is to be administered over 6 hours)
- Drops per mL = 20 (as your infusion set delivers 20 drops per mL)

This would work out at:

$$\text{Drops rate per minute} = \frac{1000}{4} \quad \frac{\times \ 20}{60}$$

Answer: 55.5 drops per minute (round up to 56)

Activity 4.3 Working out how long each infusion will last

1. 500mL of 5% dextrose is prescribed to be administered at 20 drops per minute. The administration set delivers 20 drops per mL.

- Volume in mL = 500mL (as you have a 500mL bag of fluid)
- Drops per mL = 20 (as your infusion set delivers 20 drops per mL)
- Drops per minute = 20 (as your infusion is set to deliver 20 drops per minute)

This would work out at:

$$\text{Time infusion will last (in hours)} = \frac{500}{20} \quad \frac{\times \ 20}{60}$$

Answer: 8.3 hours

2. 500mL of whole blood is prescribed to be administered at 40 drops per minute. The administration set delivers 15 drops per mL.

- Volume in mL = 500mL (as you have a 500mL bag of fluid)
- Drops per mL = 15 (as your infusion set delivers 15 drops per mL)
- Drops per minute = 40 (as your infusion is set to deliver 40 drops per minute)

This would work out at:

$$\text{Time infusion will last (in hours)} = \frac{500}{40} \times \frac{15}{60}$$

Answer: 3.125 hours

3. 100mL of Hartmann's solution is prescribed to be administered at 10 drops per minute. The administration set delivers 20 drops per mL.

- Volume in mL = 100mL (as you have a 100mL bag of fluid)
- Drops per mL = 20 (as your infusion set delivers 20 drops per mL)
- Drops per minute = 10 (as your infusion is set to deliver 10 drops per minute)

This would work out at:

$$\text{Time infusion will last (in hours)} = \frac{100}{40} \times \frac{20}{60}$$

Answer: 3.3 hours

Activity 6.2 Working out the infusion rate in drops per minute

1. If 1 litre (1L) 5% glucose is prescribed and to be administered over 8 hours, using a standard giving set delivering 20 drops per mL, what would the infusion rate be in drops per minute?

This would work out at:

$$\frac{1000 \times 20}{480 \text{ minutes}}$$

Answer: 23.6 drops per minute (round up to 24)

2. If 500mL sodium chloride is prescribed and to be administered over 2 hours, using a standard giving set delivering 20 drops per mL, what would the infusion rate be in drops per minute?

This would work out at:

$$\frac{500 \quad \times \quad 20}{120 \text{ minutes}}$$

Answer: 83.3 drops per minute (round down to 83)

3. If 1 litre (1L) 5% glucose is prescribed and to be administered over 6 hours, using a standard giving set delivering 20 drops per mL, what would the infusion rate be in drops per minute?

$$\frac{1000 \quad \times \quad 20}{360 \text{ minutes}}$$

Answer: 55.5 drops per minute (round up to 56)

References

Amoore, J. & Adamson, L. (2003). Infusion devices: characteristics, limitations and risk management. *Nursing Standard.* 17(28), 45–52.

Amoore, J. & Ingram, P. (2002). Syringe pumps and start up time. *Nursing Standard.* **15**(17), 43–45.

Boyd, C. (2013). *Medicine Management Skills for Nurses.* (3rd edn). Oxford: Wiley Blackwell.

Clayton, M. (1987). The right way to prevent medicines errors. *Registered Nurse.* **50**(30), 1.

Department of Health (DH) (2000). *An Organisation with Memory.* London: Stationery Office.

Department of Health (DH) (2011). *High Impact Intervention Number 2: Peripheral Intravenous Cannula Care bundle.* http://webarchive.nationalarchives.gov.uk/20120118164404/hcai.dh.gov.uk/files/2011/03/2011-03-14-HII-Peripheral-intravenous-cannula-bundle-FIN%E2%80%A6.pdf (Accessed 26.5.2017).

Dougherty, L. (2002). Delivery of intravenous therapy. *Nursing Standard.* **16**(16), 45–52.

Dougherty, L. (2008). Peripheral cannulation. *Nursing Standard.* **22**(52), 49–56.

Dougherty, L. & Watson, J. (2008). 'Vascular access devices' in L. Dougherty & S. Lister (eds) *The Royal Marsden Hospital Manual of Clinical Nursing Procedures* (9th edn). Oxford: Blackwell Publishing.

Drain, K.L. & Volcheck, G.W. (2001). Preventing and managing drug induced anaphylaxis. *Drug Safety.* **24**(11), 843–53.

Endacott, R., Jevon, P. & Cooper, S. (2009). *Clinical Nursing Skills: Core and Advanced.* Oxford: Oxford University Press.

Gabriel, J. (2008). Infusion therapy part two: prevention and management of complications. *Nursing Standard.* **22** (32), 41–48.

Gabriel, J., Bravery, K., Dougherty, L., Kayley, J. & Scales, K. (2005). Vascular access: indications and implications for patient care. *Nursing Standard.* **19**(26), 45–52.

Hadaway, L. & Millam, D. (2005). On the road to successful IV starts. *Nursing.* **35**, 1–14.

Hamilton, H. (2000). Selecting the correct intravenous device nursing assessment. *British Journal of Nursing.* **9**(15), 968–78.

Health and Safety Executive (HSE) (2013). *Health and Safety (Sharp Instruments in Healthcare) Regulations 2013.* HSE. London. http://www.hse.gov.uk/pubns/hsis7.pdf (Accessed 26.5.2017).

Higginson, R. (2011). Phlebitis: treatment, care and prevention. *Nursing Times.* **107**(36), 18–21.

Hindley, G. (2004) Infection control in peripheral cannulae. *Nursing Standard.* **18**(27), 37–40.

Ingram, P. & Lavery, I. (2005). Peripheral intravenous therapy: key risks and implications for practice. *Nursing Standard.* **19**(46), 55–64.

Jackson, A. (1998). Infection control: a battle in vein infusion phlebitis. *Nursing Times.* **94**(4), 68–71.

Lavery, I. (2010). Infection control in IV therapy: a review of the chain of infection. *British Journal of Nursing.* **19**(19), S6–S14.

Lavery, I. & Ingram, P. (2008). Safe practice in intravenous medicines administration. *Nursing Standard.* **22**(46), 44–47.

Loveday, H.P., Wilson, J.A., Pratt, R.J., Golsorkhi, M., Tinle, A., Bak, A., Browne, J., Prieto, J. & Wilcox, M. (2014). epic 3: National Evidence-Based Guidelines for Preventing Healthcare-Associated Infections in NHS Hospitals in England. *Journal of Hospital Infection.* http://www.his.org.uk/files/3113/8693/4808/epic3_National_Evidence-Based_Guidelines_for_Preventing_HCAI_in_NHSE.pdf (Accessed 26.5.2017).

McCall, R. & Tankersley, C.M. (2008). *Phlebotomy Essentials Workbook.* (4th edn). Philadelphia: Lippincott and Williams. P

McCallum, L. & Higgins, D. (2012). Care of peripheral venous cannula sites. *Nursing Times.* **108**(34), 35.

Medical Devices Agency (2000). *Single use medical devices: Implications and Consequences of Reuse.* MDA DB (04). London: The Stationery Office.

Nair, M. & Peate, I. (2013). *Fundamentals of Applied Pathophysiology: An Essential Guide for Nursing & Healthcare.* Chichester: Wiley Blackwell.

National Patient Safety Agency (NPSA) (2006). *Right patient, right blood. Safer Practice Notice.* 14. London: NPSA.

National Patient Safety Agency (NPSA) (2007). *Promoting safer use of injectable medicines.* http://www.nrls.npsa.nhs.uk/resources/?entryid45=59812 (Accessed 26.5.2017).

National Patient Safety Agency (NPSA) (2009). *Safety in doses: Improving the use of medicines in the NHS*. London: NPSA.

Nursing and Midwifery Council (NMC) (2008). *Standards for Medicines Management*. London: NMC.

Nursing and Midwifery Council (NMC) (2015). *The Code: Professional standards and behaviour for nurses and midwives*. London: NMC. http://www.nmc.org.uk/globalassets/sitedocuments/nmc-publications/revised-new-nmc-code.pdf (Accessed 26.5.2017).

O'Brien, M., Spires, A. & Andrews, K. (2011). *Introduction to Medicines Management in Nursing*. Exeter: Learning Matters.

O'Hanlon, S., Glenn, R. & Hazler, B. (2008). Delivering intravenous therapy in the community setting. *Nursing Standard*. **22**(31), 44–48.

Reis, P.E. (2009). Pharmacological interventions to treat phlebitis, systematic review. *Journal of Infusion Nursing*. **32**(2), 74–79.

Richardson, R. (2008). *Clinical skills for student nurses – theory, practice and reflection*. Exeter: Reflect Press.

Rowley, S. (2001). Aseptic Non Touch Technique. *Nursing Times*. **97**(7), 6.

Royal College of Nursing (RCN) (2010). *Standards for Infusion Therapy*. (3rd edn.). London: Royal College of Nursing.

Scales, K. (2005). Vascular access: a guide to peripheral venous cannulation. *Nursing Standard*. **19**(49), 48–52.

Scales, K. (2008). 'Anatomy and physiology related to intravenous therapy' in L. Dougherty & J. Lamb (eds). *Intravenous Therapy in Nursing Practice*. (2nd edn). Oxford: Blackwell Publishing.

Tortora, G. & Derrickson, B. (2011). *Principles of Anatomy and Physiology*. (11th edn). Chichester: Wiley Blackwell.

Ung, L., Cook, S., Edwards, B., Hocking, L., Osmond, F. & Buttergieg, H. (2002). Peripheral intravenous cannulation in nursing: performance predictors. *Journal of Infusion Nursing*. **25**(3), 189–95.

Weinstein, S. & Hagle, M. (2014). *Plumer's principles and practice of infusion therapy*. (9th edn). Philadelphia: Lippincott, Williams and Wilkins.

Whyte, A. (2001). Well Equipped? *Nursing Times*. **97**(42), 22–23.

Wilson, J. (2001). *Infection Control in Clinical Practice*. (2nd edn). London: Balliere Tindall.

Workman, B. (1999). Peripheral intravenous therapy management. *Nursing Standard*. **14**(4), 53–60.

Index